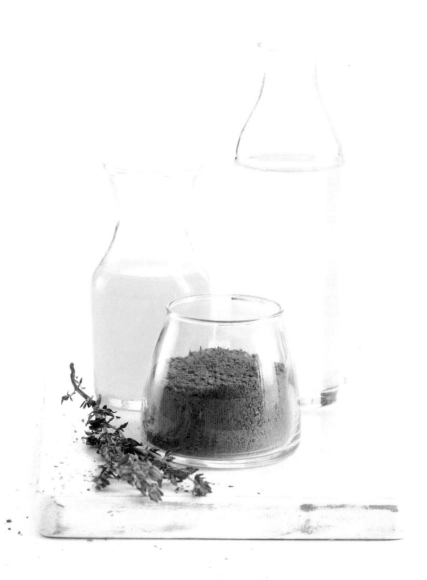

Editorial production team leader: Crystel Jobin-Gagnon
Graphic production team leader: Marie-Christine Langlois
Production coordinator: Marjorie Lajoie
Culinary content manager: Catherine Pelletier
Authors: Benoit Boudreau and Richard Houde
Chefs: Benoit Boudreau and Richard Houde
Writers: Miléna Babin, Pascale Hubert, Annie Lavoie, Fernanda Machado Gonçalves
and Raphaële St-Laurent Pelletier
Writer researcher: Isabelle Chabot
Copy editors: Marilou Cloutier and Corinne Dallain
Production assistants: Edmonde Barry, Catherine Mathis and Nancy Morel
Graphic designers: Sonia Barbeau, Sheila Basque, Marie-Chloë G. Barrette,
Karyne Ouellet and Claudia Renaud
Food stylist supervisor: Christine Morin
Food stylists: Louise Bouchard, Laurie Collin, Maude Grimard, Carly Harvey, Christine
Morin and Julie Morin
Photography supervisor: Marie-Ève Lévesque
Photographers: Mélanie Blais, Rémy Germain and Martin Houde
Photographer and videographer: Tony Davidson
Imaging processing and photography calibration specialist: Yves Vaillancourt
Collaborators: Jean-Christophe Blanchet, Lucie Lévesque-Pageau and Pub Photo
Translation: Edgar

Legal deposit: 4th quarter 2018
Bibliothèque et Archives nationales du Québec
National Library and Archives of Canada

ISBN: 9782896586615

(Original edition: ISBN 978-2-89658-611-0, Éditions Pratico-pratiques inc.,
Québec)

Gouvernement du Québec – Refundable Tax Credit for Book Publishing program –
Gestion SODEC

1685 Talbot Boulevard, Québec, QC G2N 0C6
Tel.: 418-877-0259
Toll-free: 1-866-882-0091
Fax: 418-780-1716
www.pratico-pratiques.com

Comments and suggestions: info@pratico-pratiques.com

400 CALORIES *or less!*

Enjoy food, guilt-free

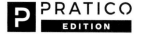
PRATICO EDITION

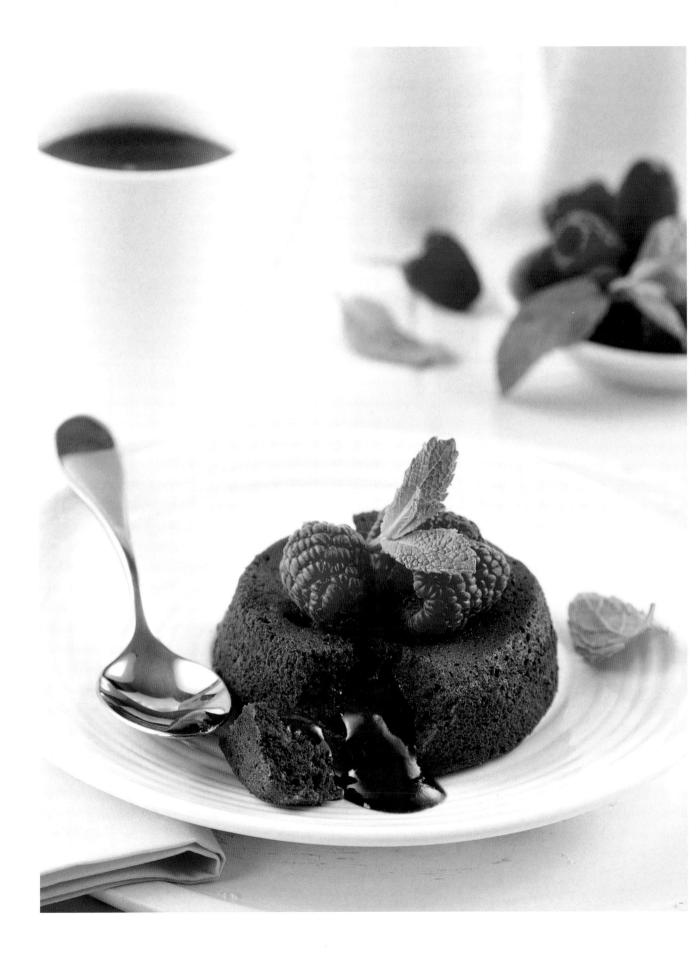

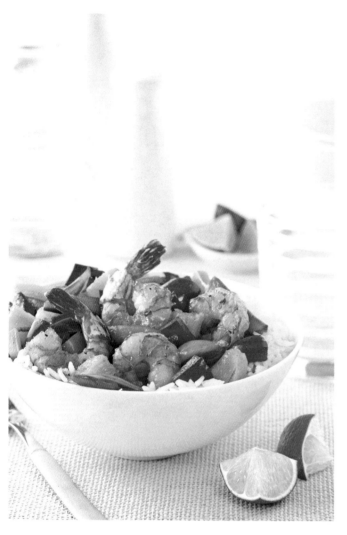

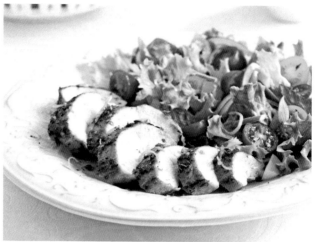

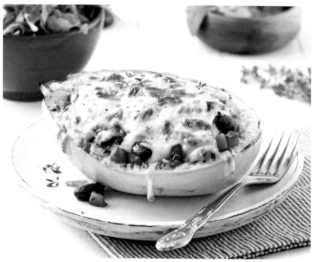

Table of Contents

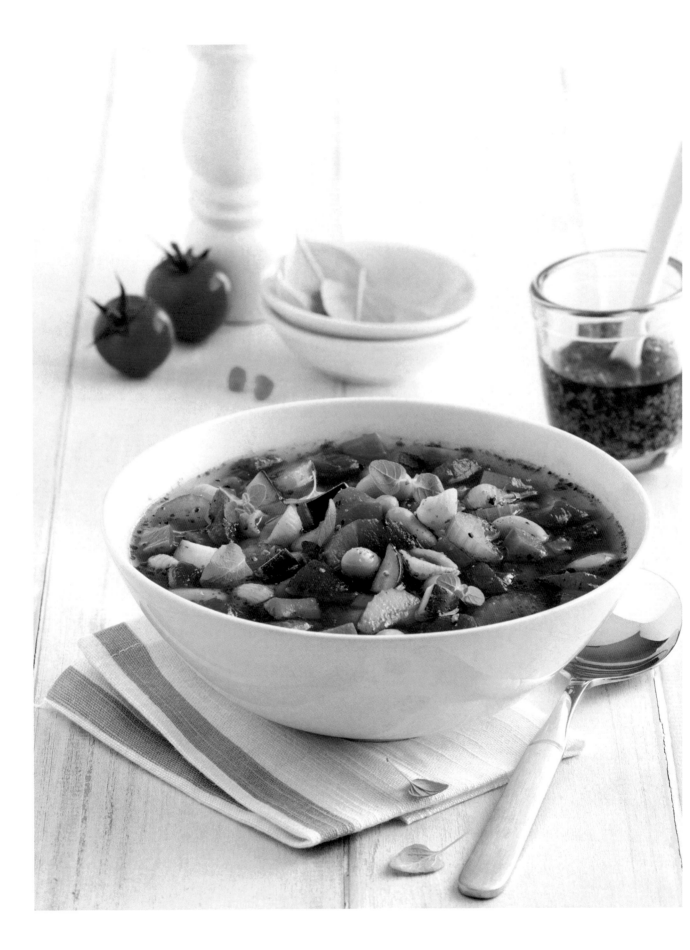

Eat well, without limiting yourself

What a pleasure it is to eat!

For all of us epicureans, food is all about discovering flavours from both near and far. Tasting new and delicious dishes, experimenting with culinary trends… What a joy! Who wants to ignore their gut when it comes to trying such appetizing pleasures?

Nevertheless, we all know that food has a direct influence on our quality of life, and are aware of the importance of eating better, in a more balanced way. But dieters beware—eating a balanced diet does not mean depriving yourself! The trick? Choose foods that are healthy, nutritious, filling and low in fat to create low-calorie, highly delectable meals.

This book is proof that it's possible to treat yourself with dishes that contain no more than 400 calories. Whether you're looking to lose some weight or just maintain your current weight, this book is for you! You'll find over 100 different delicious recipes, each with 400 calories or less for mains and less than 200 calories for desserts.

Food that's mouth-watering but guilt-free!

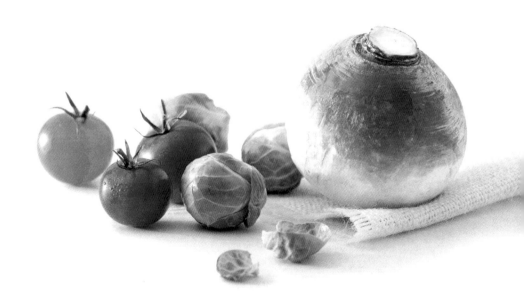

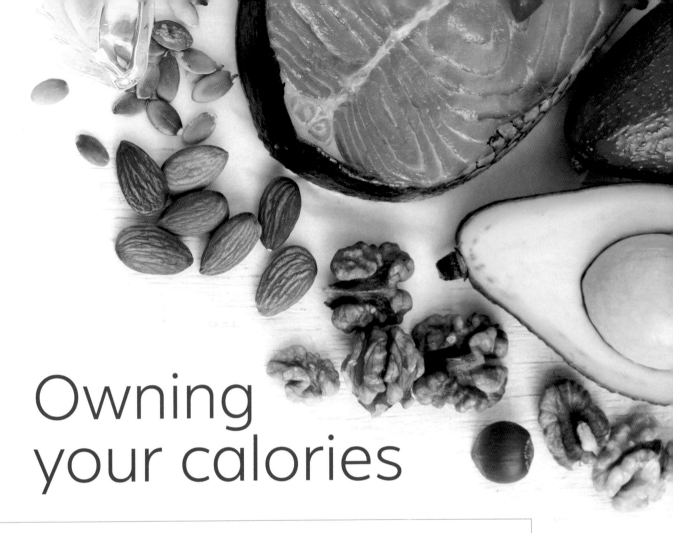

Owning your calories

Whether you've made peace with calories or declared war on them, they are a necessary part of life. Our bodies need a certain number of calories each day in order to function properly, so it's important to learn how to handle them.

But what exactly is a calorie? Stripped to the bare essentials, a calorie is a unit that measures how much energy our bodies take from the food we eat.

Calories can be found in carbohydrates, proteins and lipids (fats). There are 4 calories per gram in these first two nutrient types, and 9 calories (more than double!) in lipids. Alcoholic beverages provide 7 calories per gram, but these calories are considered "empty" because they have no nutritional value. The daily needs of our bodies vary depending on sex, age and activity level. For example, a woman between 31 and 50 years old needs 1,800 to 2,250 calories per day depending on how active she is. A man in the same age range needs to consume 2,350 to 2,900 calories per day. And basal metabolism decreases with age, which means that your body needs fewer calories later in life.

In the following pages, we'll tell you about pitfalls to avoid, bust some myths, give you some tips and tricks to remember, and provide sound data to help you better understand calories.

Pictures: Shutterstock.

Why do we put on weight?

Calories are the number one enemy of so many people who struggle with their weight. But are they really the sole culprit when it comes to extra pounds? Absolutely not.

Weight gain can be brought on by several factors. It generally occurs when your body absorbs more calories than it actually needs to function properly. The surplus of calories then gets stored as fat in fat cells. The situation can be even worse if you have a sedentary lifestyle or if you aren't active enough to burn the extra calories. The small amount of energy that you spend, compared to the calories you consume while eating and drinking, creates an unbalance that leads to excess weight.

Certain harmful eating habits are also to blame. Skipping meals like breakfast is one of the most common, but it's important to know that missing a meal makes metabolism slow down in an effort to save energy. The result? Your body stocks up on fat. And when you run out of energy before your next meal, you wind up compensating by absent-mindedly snacking on whatever you have on hand.

Finally, other factors such as metabolism, genes, stress, family difficulties, professional concerns and even diets that are too strict can also be at fault.

Does lowering your calorie intake trim fat?

You can't go without a certain number of calories. They are the fuel that keeps your body's vital functions working the way they should. However, it is our responsibility to avoid accumulating more than the daily recommended amount and to remain active at the same time—this is the true key to staying thin!

To manage your weight, the formula is simple. The more you move, the more energy you spend, the more you burn the calories you don't need. Ideally, you should exercise for 30 to 60 minutes every day. If going to the gym or shaking to the rhythm of Zumba isn't your cup of tea, take a walk after work (equipped with a pedometer), run your errands on rollerblades, garden, swim, play with your kids, hop on the stationary bike, shovel the snow, etc.

Managing your calories shouldn't be rocket science. Eat slowly and concentrate on your food. Avoid watching TV, reading or doing any other distracting activity. Listen to your body and respect it when it tells you you're hungry or you're satiated.

Food combinations and dairy products

We often hear that combining two starches leads to weight gain, but this isn't the case. It's not so much eating bread with pasta or rice that you should limit. Instead, make sure to respect a certain balance between the energy provided by these foods and the energy that your body uses. Remembering a few simple tips can help you achieve this energy balance: serve yourself a smaller portion of pasta if you want a slice of bread, choose more filling whole grain carbs and watch what you spread on your bread (cheese, butter...).

Similarly, eating gratins isn't harmful if you don't overdo it. Adding about 30 to 50 g (1 to 1½ oz.) of skim milk cheese per serving will also help you increase your consumption of dairy products. Dairy provides us with a few of our essential vitamins and minerals and satiates the appetite, which is a big plus for controlling our weight.

Instead of banning dairy products, take the advice from *Canada's Food Guide* and consume two or three servings a day. As a general rule, one serving is equal to 250 ml (1 cup) of milk or 175 g (¾ cup) of yogourt. Try anything made with skim milk. With 0.2 g of fat, skim milk contains 41 calories fewer per 250 ml than 2% milk, which also contains 25 times more fat (5.1 g). Replace cream with milk or use cheese with a strong flavour so that you can use a little less.

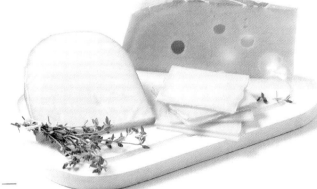

Did you say "light"?

You should always be vigilant and inspect the ingredients list and the nutrition facts label before filling your grocery cart with "light" products. Products labelled "light" or "low-fat" are not necessarily better for your figure. In many cases, these products only have 11% fewer calories than the regular version. And the fat is often replaced by sugar or sugar substitutes that nurture your sweet tooth. According to some studies, these artificial sweeteners might even increase hunger cravings. So make sure to compare the caloric value of the light and regular versions before making your choice.

What's more, these light products can even play a role in making us gain weight because we tend to eat more (up to 35% more!) without feeling an ounce of guilt. Take it from us: instead of tempting yourself with a double dose of supposedly light food, make a habit of enjoying a smaller portion of the real stuff.

Read the labels!

Reading labels is the most effective way to identify high calorie foods and only takes a split second. It's a baby step that can do a lot to help you maintain a healthy weight.

The Nutrition Facts table on the back of prepackaged food is regulated by Health Canada and is based on an average intake of 2,000 calories per day. As a general rule, this number meets the calorie needs of an average-sized woman who is moderately active, an average sized man who is sedentary or an adolescent who is glued to a computer all day. Of course, that number has to be adjusted according to a person's build, age and individual activity level.

For each food, the calories are indicated for a specific serving size. Whenever possible when you compare products, take into account the weight (g) or volume (ml) of each given serving size. Furthermore, if you consume more than the suggested serving size, you should re-evaluate how many calories you're actually taking in accordingly. For example, if 160 calories are calculated for a 175 g (¾ cup) serving of yogourt, and you eat twice that amount, you are actually consuming 320 calories. You should also check the fibre percentage, listed in the carbohydrate section—the higher, the better. If the fibre content is high, you know that the food you're coveting has unparalleled satiating power. If it's low, you'll be more likely to fill up on it to alleviate those hunger pangs.

Lastly, you should always read over the ingredients list of each food item, including the additives. Is sugar at the top of the list? That product probably contains added sugar. Beware the empty calories!

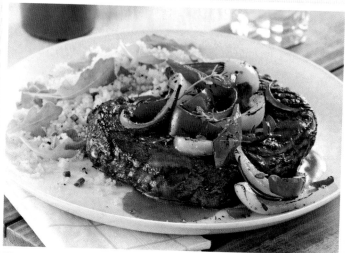

And what about meat?

Animal proteins are part of a balanced diet, but some are more adapted to our slender goals than others!

Although red meat contains several nutritional elements (iron, zinc, B complex vitamins), it's quite high in saturated fat and cholesterol. The visible fat alone of a 100 g serving of beef adds 100 calories to the portion. You're better off removing it! Choosing lean cuts and cooking methods that don't require much extra fat (think oven, grill, wok) can be a great alternative to giving up red meat entirely. According to *Canada's Food Guide*, eating one 75 g (2½ oz.) serving of red meat is enough to feel satiated.

As for lean proteins, white meat (poultry, pork, veal) has fewer calories and is perfect for treating yourself to a variety of tasty meats without putting on weight. For example, 100 g of chicken breast contains 173 calories, and 100 g of pork tenderloin contains 162. Compare that with the same portion of lean ground beef, which has 252 calories. The choice is up to you!

Winning tips for losing weight!

Dropping pounds without depriving yourself is possible. How? By integrating healthy habits into your routine. Try it for yourself!

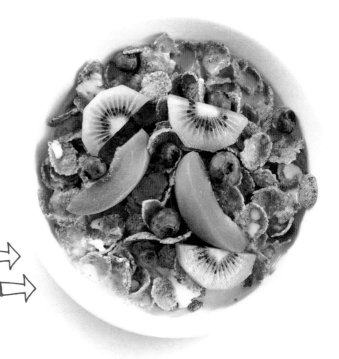

- **Eat a balanced breakfast** by combining at least three of the four groups listed in *Canada's Food Guide* (e.g., fruits, grains, dairy products) and by making sure that you're getting at least 15 g of protein. If you fill up on energy in the morning, you'll have an easier time curbing your appetite. A healthy breakfast will ward off the munchies and sugar cravings between meals, which prevents potential weight gain.

- **Opt for healthy snacks** that contain between 2 and 5 g of protein and between 100 and 200 calories. They should also come from at least two of the four groups listed in *Canada's Food Guide*. To help your body feel satiated, combine a carbohydrate with a protein. Try yogourt and fruit, or raw vegetables and a piece of cheese.

- **Consume more fruits and vegetables.** Fresh produce is nutritious, low in calories and rich in fibre. Remember that the daily recommended fibre intake is 25 g for women and 38 g for men. Fibre-rich foods help you feel satisfied more quickly, meaning you'll eat less during and in between meals. The recap: more fibre equals fewer calories at the end of the day and less weight on the scale over time.

- **Manage your portions.** Don't worry—you can still be a part of the clean plate club! Just choose a smaller plate size with an interior diameter of about 20 cm, or 8 in. Then divvy up its contents. Reserve half of the plate for colourful vegetables, a quarter for protein (meat, eggs, etc.) and another quarter for whole grains (pasta, rice, etc.). By reducing your portions by 10 to 20%, you'll eat less and lower your calorie intake without even noticing.

- **Watch what you drink.** Fruit punch, carbonated drinks and other sugary cocktails are not ideal. Taking gulps of these empty calories won't relieve hunger. Biting into an actual apple (72 calories) instead of drinking juice from the same fruit (119 calories for 250 ml) will satisfy hunger cravings without the added guilt. Three cheers for healthy snacking!

- **Go easy on alcohol.** Every gram of alcohol contains 7 calories. So drinking that little glass of port wine, just 60 ml (¼ cup) for a light aperitif, means you've just downed 90 calories! Plus, alcohol masks satiety signals and whets the appetite, so it can increase the number of calories you consume during your next meal.

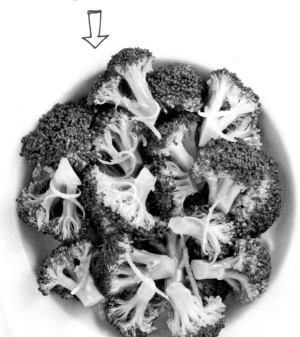

Myth or reality?

Some myths die hard. We're here to dispel a few popular beliefs!

- **Drinking water makes you lose weight.**
  Water definitely doesn't contain calories, and it keeps us hydrated—but it has no direct effect on weight loss. However, drinking large amounts of water often relieves the urge to snack, and that's always a good thing! Plus, if you work out, it's good to know that your body burns fat faster when you're properly hydrated.

- **Dense bread contains more calories.** Made of just water, flour and salt, bread is low in fat (about 1% depending on the type of bread). But it does contain a lot of carbohydrates (about 60%). Whole grain breads with a denser texture are rich in fibre. Unlike white breads made with refined flour, whole grain breads quickly satisfy your hunger.

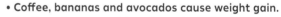

- **Coffee, bananas and avocados cause weight gain.**
  We'll say it once and for all: no single food has the power to make you gain or lose weight. Plain black coffee only has 3 calories. But things get complicated when we give in to specialty coffee drinks like mochas, vanilla lattes and cappuccinos. The caloric density of these treats can spike up to 190 calories per cup. Similarly, occasionally eating fruits that have a high fat content, like avocados or bananas, won't ruin your waistline. Despite having 300 calories (comparable to 30 ml or 2 tbsp of oil), avocados are a good source of monounsaturated fat and contain fibre. As for bananas, they might have 100 to 120 calories, but you would have to eat 30 to 35 of them before gaining about one pound (3,500 calories).

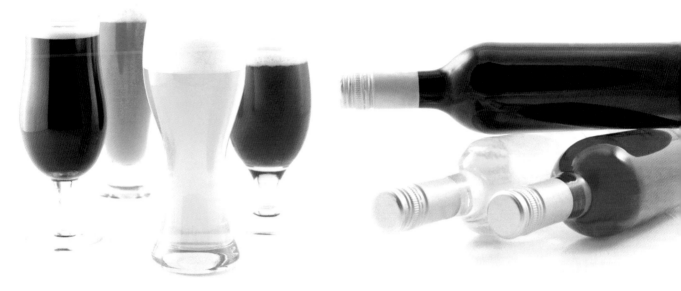

Choose wisely—compare the calories!

Lower calorie choice	Calories	Higher calorie choice	Calories
1 single-serve tub (15 ml) of 2% milk creamer	8	1 single-serve tub (15 ml) of 10% creamer	18
30 ml (2 tbsp) of dairy blend for cooking (5%)	29	30 ml (2 tbsp) of cooking cream (15%)	50
250 ml (1 cup) of skim milk	88	250 ml (1 cup) of 2% milk	129
175 g (¾ cup) of plain yogourt (0%)	60	175 g (¾ cup) of plain yogourt (2%)	90
50 g (1½ oz.) of skim milk cheddar cheese	141	50 g (1½ oz.) of regular cheddar cheese	203
1 slice (35 g) of whole wheat bread	90	1 slice (35 g) of white bread	91
100 g of phyllo dough	299	100 g of puff pastry	551
250 ml (8 oz.) of beer	108	250 ml (8 oz.) of red wine	212

Sides that pile on the pounds!

Side Dish	Calories
125 ml (½ cup) of boiled green beans	23
125 ml (½ cup) of cooked sliced carrots	29
125 ml (½ cup) of mashed potatoes, made with 2% milk	90
125 ml (½ cup) of cooked white rice	109
125 ml (½ cup) of cooked fettuccine noodles, made with white flour	117
1 medium-sized (173 g) plain baked potato (with skin)	161

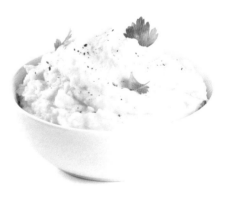

Hearty Soups

Hearty soups are the perfect solution for a quick dinner because they can be made in the blink of an eye. What's more, just one bowl can be a great source of vitamins and provides a generous dose of comfort. Try any of these recipes prepared with a vegetable, poultry, meat or seafood base for a satisfying meal you can indulge in.

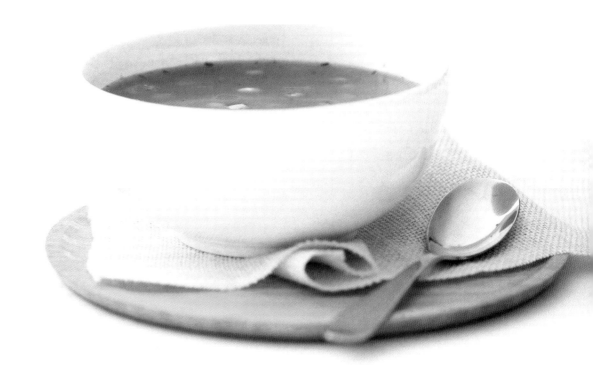

Vietnamese Shrimp Soup

125 g (¼ lb) rice noodles

15 ml (1 tbsp) olive oil

1 stem lemongrass

750 ml (3 cups) vegetable stock

15 ml (1 tbsp) ginger, minced

10 ml (2 tsp) garlic, minced

4 to 5 drops fish sauce
(nuoc mam)

Hot chili pepper to taste,
chopped

1 carrot, chopped

2 celery stalks, chopped

12 baby bok choy heads

16 medium shrimp
(31-40 count), raw and peeled

30 ml (2 tbsp) fresh
cilantro, chopped

Prep time **30 minutes**

Cook time **13 minutes**

Serves **4**

PER SERVING	
Calories	184
Protein	10 g
Fat	2 g
Carbohydrates	33 g
Fibre	3 g
Iron	2 mg
Calcium	169 mg
Sodium	930 mg

1. Prepare the noodles according to the instructions on the packaging. Drain and drizzle with olive oil. Stir and set aside.

2. Cut the lemongrass stem in half lengthwise.

3. Place the vegetable stock in a pot and bring to a boil. Add the lemongrass, ginger, garlic, fish sauce and hot pepper. Let simmer over medium heat for 8 to 10 minutes.

4. Remove the lemongrass. Add the carrot, celery, baby bok choy, shrimp and noodles. Bring to a boil again. Let simmer for 5 minutes, until the vegetables are tender.

5. Add the cilantro before serving. Let infuse for 1 minute before distributing the soup into bowls.

Did you know?

Eating shrimp is good for your heart and body!
Whether it's northern, black tiger or another variety, shrimp is rich in protein and low in calories: 100 g of shrimp contains 17 g of protein and provides between 95 and 110 calories, depending on the species. It's the perfect food for people who are watching their weight! Shrimp is also packed with vitamins and minerals (vitamins B3 and B12, phosphorus, copper, selenium, magnesium…) and low in saturated fat, and contains the omega-3 fatty acids your body requires to keep your heart healthy. Did you know that one serving of 100 g makes up for 80% of your daily omega-3 needs? And remember that although shrimp is high in cholesterol, that number actually has very little effect on your blood cholesterol levels.

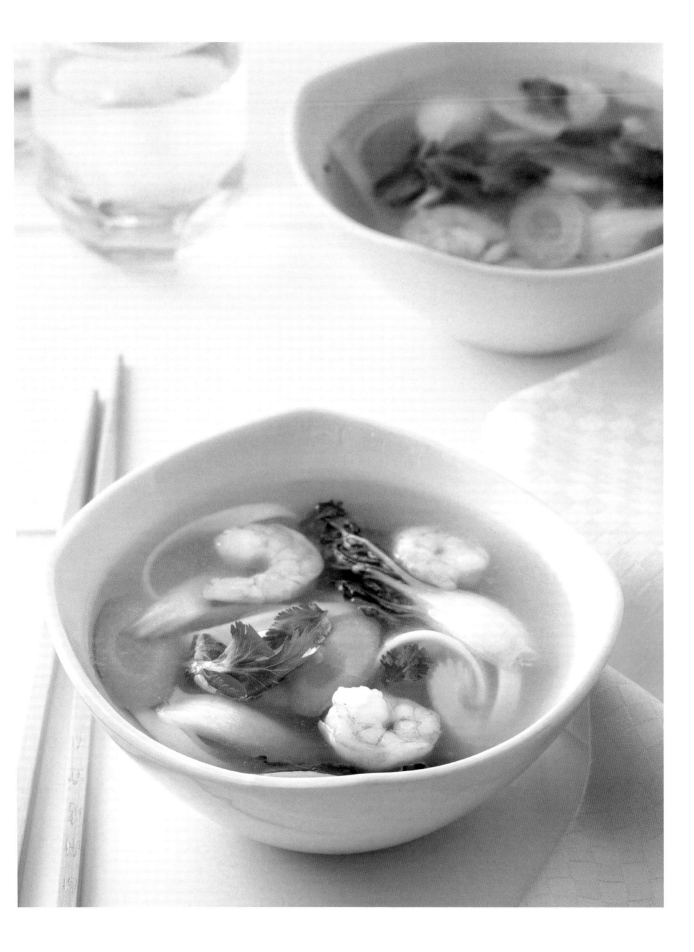

Chicken and Potato Soup

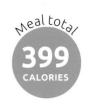

Meal total
399
CALORIES

30 ml (2 tbsp) butter

700 g (1 ½ lb) frozen diced vegetable mix, thawed and drained

8 slices precooked bacon, chopped

3 potatoes, diced

1 litre (4 cups) chicken stock

500 ml (2 cups) cooked chicken, shredded

60 ml (¼ cup) fresh parsley, chopped

Salt and pepper to taste

Prep time **15 minutes**

Cook time **20 minutes**

Serves **4**

PER SERVING	
Calories	399
Protein	32 g
Fat	13 g
Carbohydrates	40 g
Fibre	8 g
Iron	3 mg
Calcium	140 mg
Sodium	1,207 mg

1. Melt the butter in a pot over medium heat. Cook the diced vegetables and bacon for 2 to 3 minutes.

2. Add the potatoes and stock. Cover and let simmer over medium-low heat for 15 to 20 minutes.

3. Add the chicken and parsley. Cook for another 5 minutes. Season with salt and pepper.

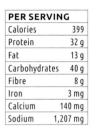

Did you know?

Potatoes are rich in vitamins

Did you know that a medium, unpeeled potato contains more iron than a cup (250 ml) of fresh spinach and more vitamin C than three peaches? And if you think that a potato will "make you fat", keep in mind that there are more calories in a bowl of white rice.

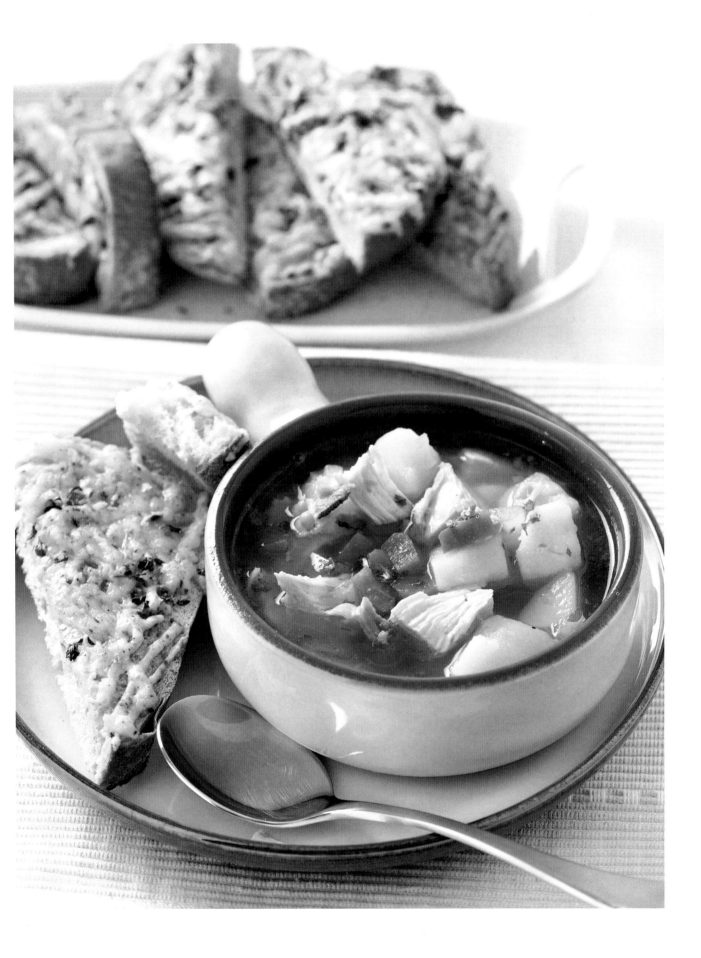

Slow Cooker Lentil Soup

2 carrots

½ butternut squash

3 potatoes

2 celery stalks

1 onion

1 leek

3 Italian tomatoes

1 litre (4 cups) vegetable stock (low-sodium)

A few sprigs thyme, chopped

1 bay leaf

250 ml (1 cup) dry green lentils

15 ml (1 tbsp) garlic, minced

5 ml (1 tsp) turmeric

Salt and pepper to taste

500 ml (2 cups) kale, chopped

Prep time **20 minutes**

Cook time on low **7 hours**

Serves **4**

PER SERVING	
Calories	390
Protein	21 g
Fat	2 g
Carbohydrates	77 g
Fibre	14 g
Iron	8 mg
Calcium	195 mg
Sodium	220 mg

1. Dice the carrots, squash, potatoes, celery, onion, leek and tomatoes.

2. Place the vegetables, stock, herbs, lentils, garlic and turmeric in a slow cooker. Season with salt and pepper, and stir.

3. Cover and cook on low for 6 to 7 hours.

4. Add the kale and stir. Cover and cook for 1 more hour.

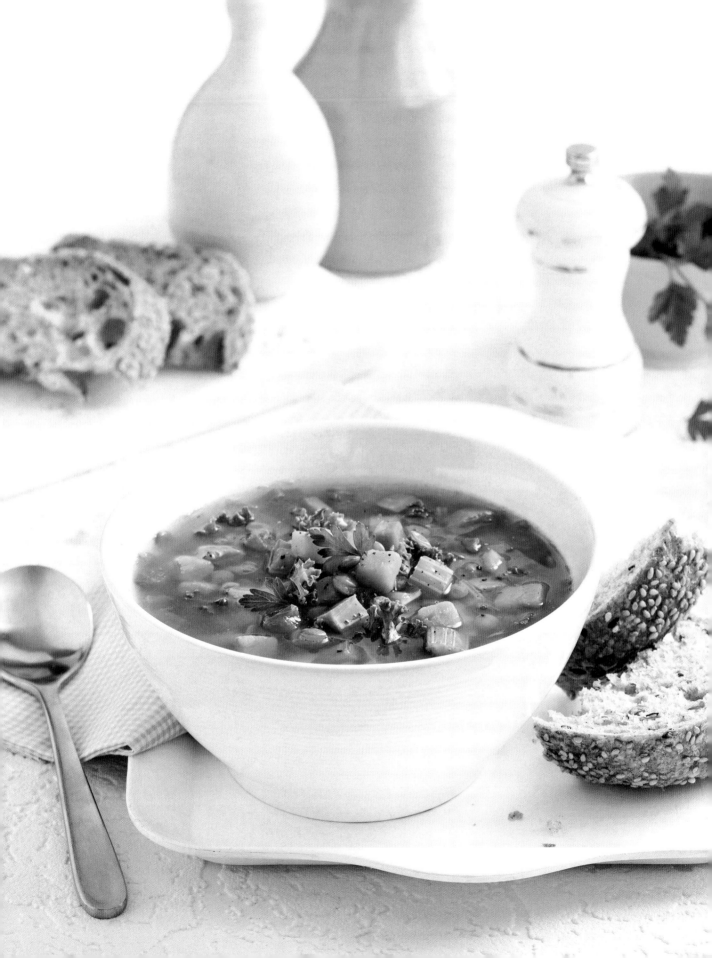

Minestrone Soup

15 ml (1 tbsp) olive oil

1 onion, diced

15 ml (1 tbsp) garlic, minced

2 carrots, diced

2 celery stalks, diced

1.5 litre (6 cups) vegetable stock (low-sodium)

1 can (540 ml) diced tomatoes

1 can (540 ml) white beans, rinsed and drained

250 ml (1 cup) small pasta shells

2 small zucchinis, diced

Salt and pepper to taste

15 ml (1 tbsp) basil pesto

Prep time **20 minutes**

Cook time **22 minutes**

Serves **4**

PER SERVING	
Calories	357
Protein	16 g
Fat	6 g
Carbohydrates	63 g
Fibre	11 g
Iron	6 mg
Calcium	183 mg
Sodium	486 mg

1. Heat the oil in a pot over medium heat. Cook the onion, garlic, carrots and celery for 2 minutes.

2. Add the stock and tomatoes. Bring to a boil, and then simmer for 10 minutes on low heat.

3. Add the beans, shells and zucchinis. Season with salt and pepper. Bring to a boil once again, and then let simmer for 10 to 12 minutes.

4. Add the pesto and stir before serving.

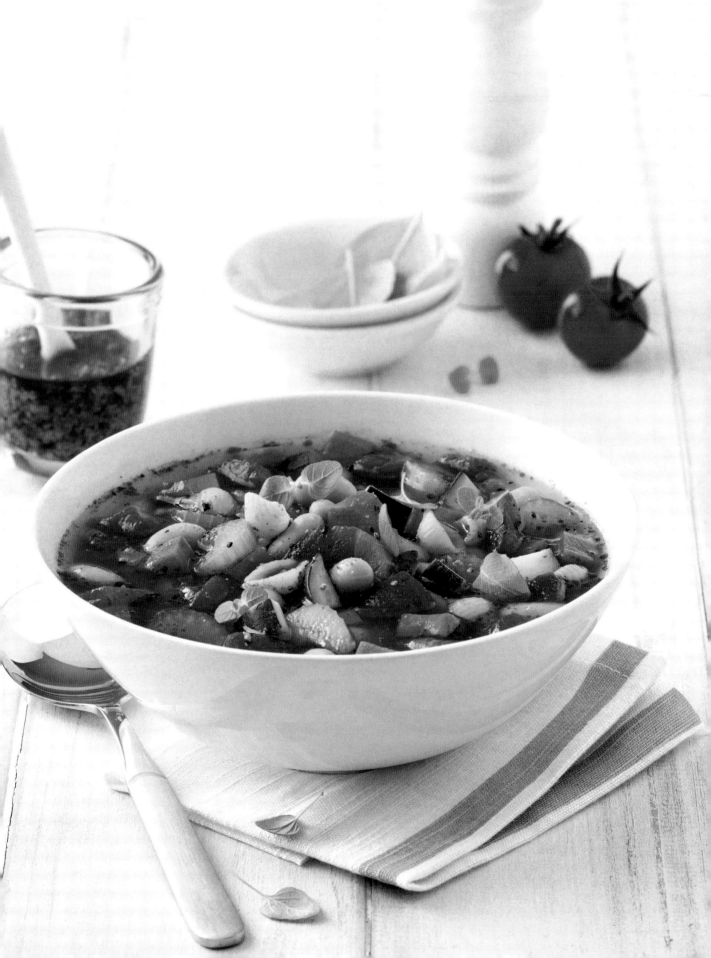

Ham and Corn Chowder

30 ml (2 tbsp) canola oil

2 onions, chopped

3 celery stalks, chopped

60 ml (¼ cup) flour

1 litre (4 cups) chicken stock

1 litre (4 cups) milk

1 smoked ham, 375 g
(about ¾ lb), diced

1 bay leaf

1 sprig thyme

Salt and pepper to taste

250 ml (1 cup) corn
kernels, fresh or frozen

375 ml (1 ½ cups) potatoes,
diced

250 ml (1 cup) sweet potatoes,
diced

Prep time **25 minutes**

Cook time **47 minutes**

Serves **6**

1. Heat the oil in a pot over medium heat. Sauté the onions with the celery for 2 to 3 minutes.

2. Stir in the flour and then pour in the chicken stock, whisking.

3. Add the milk, ham and herbs. Season with salt and pepper. Bring to a boil. Cover and let simmer for 30 minutes over low heat.

4. Add the corn and both kinds of potatoes. Cook for 15 to 20 minutes, until the vegetables are tender.

PER SERVING	
Calories	309
Protein	19 g
Fat	12 g
Carbohydrates	32 g
Fibre	3 g
Iron	2 mg
Calcium	240 mg
Sodium	1,400 mg

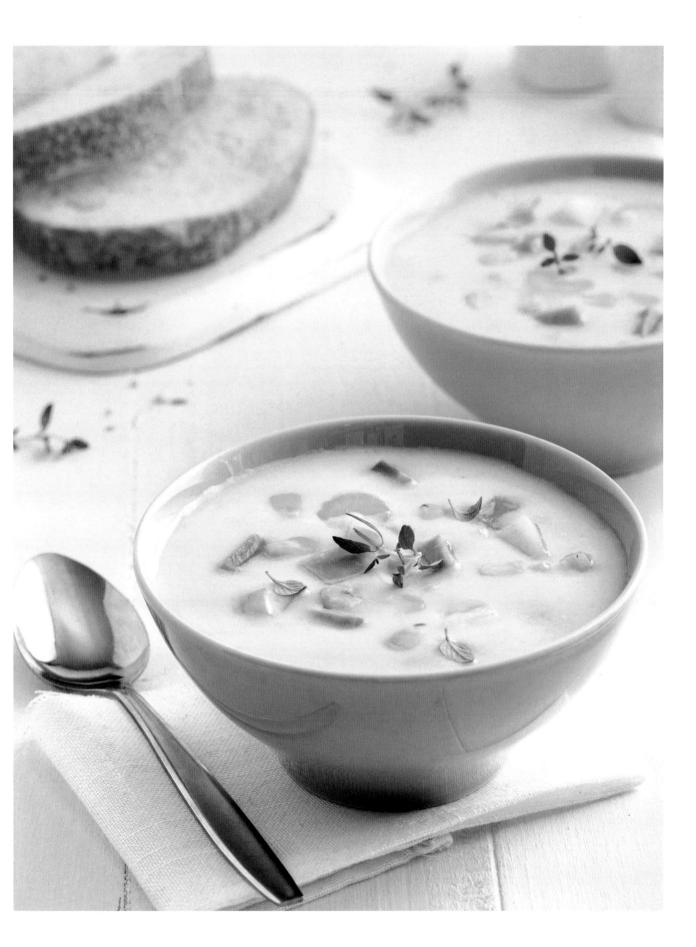

Chicken Noodle Soup

15 ml (1 tbsp) butter

1 onion, diced

1.5 litre (6 cups) chicken stock

1 to 2 carrots, diced

1 whole celery stalk (including leaves), diced

375 ml (1 ½ cups) large egg noodles

500 ml (2 cups) cooked chicken, shredded

Prep time **15 minutes**

Cook time **20 minutes**

Serves **4**

PER SERVING	
Calories	265
Protein	30 g
Fat	6 g
Carbohydrates	22 g
Fibre	2 g
Iron	1 mg
Calcium	43 mg
Sodium	1,518 mg

1. Melt the butter in a pot over medium heat. Cook the onion for a few minutes.

2. Add the stock and vegetables. Cook for 10 minutes.

3. Add the noodles and cooked chicken. Cook for another 10 minutes.

Did you know?

Chicken is even leaner than we think

Chicken meat is extra-lean. Without the skin, one serving of 100 g of roasted chicken breast has barely 2.1 g of fat, which is the equivalent of less than one teaspoon (5 ml) of butter. In comparison, the same quantity of extra-lean ground beef contains 7.7 g of fat. In addition to providing essential vitamins and minerals, chicken is high in protein (33 g for 100 g of chicken breast) and contains a high amount of amino acids. The dark meat in chicken (leg) is twice as rich in iron as the white meat (breast). Still, if you're watching the amount of fat in your food, remember that white meat is a better option since it contains less fat and more protein.

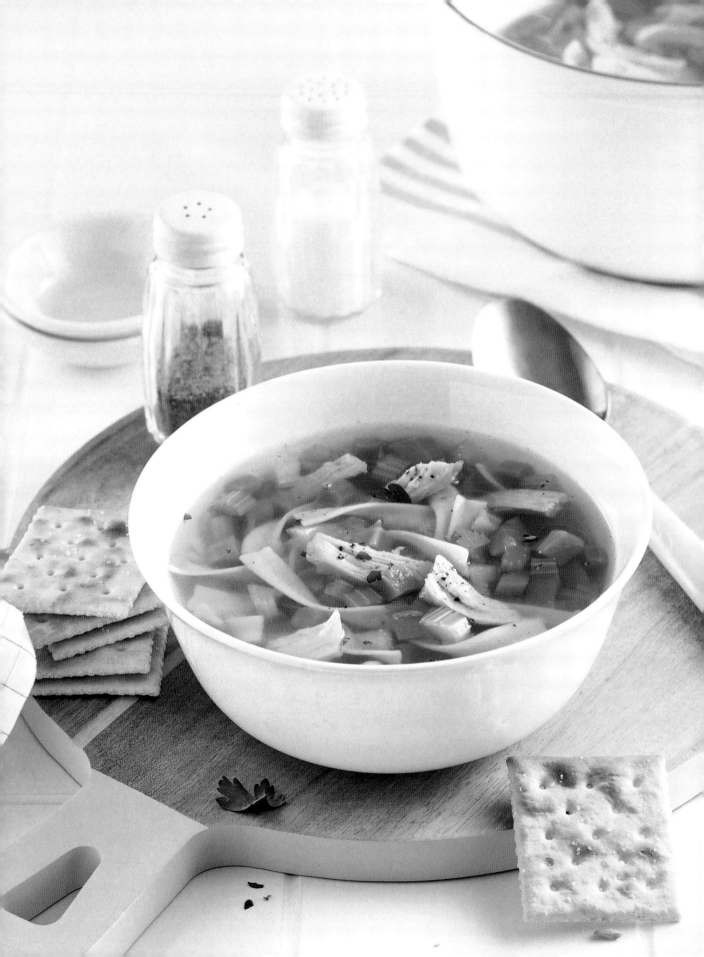

Broccoli Cheese Soup

60 ml (¼ cup) butter

1 onion, chopped

10 ml (2 tsp) minced garlic

60 ml (¼ cup) flour

750 ml (3 cups) chicken stock (no salt added)

375 ml (1 ½ cups) shredded cheddar cheese

1 broccoli, cut into small florets

180 ml (¾ cup) dairy blend for cooking (5%)

Salt and pepper to taste

Prep time **15 minutes**

Cook time **5 minutes**

Serves **4**

PER SERVING	
Calories	393
Protein	16 g
Fat	30 g
Carbohydrates	16 g
Fibre	1 g
Iron	1 mg
Calcium	353 mg
Sodium	951 mg

1. Melt the butter in a pot over medium heat. Cook the onion and garlic for 1 to 2 minutes.

2. Stir in the flour and then pour in the chicken stock. Bring to a boil, whisking.

3. Add the cheddar and stir until melted.

4. Add the broccoli and dairy blend for cooking. Season with salt and pepper. Bring to a boil and cook for 3 to 5 minutes.

5. Use an immersion blender to mix until smooth.

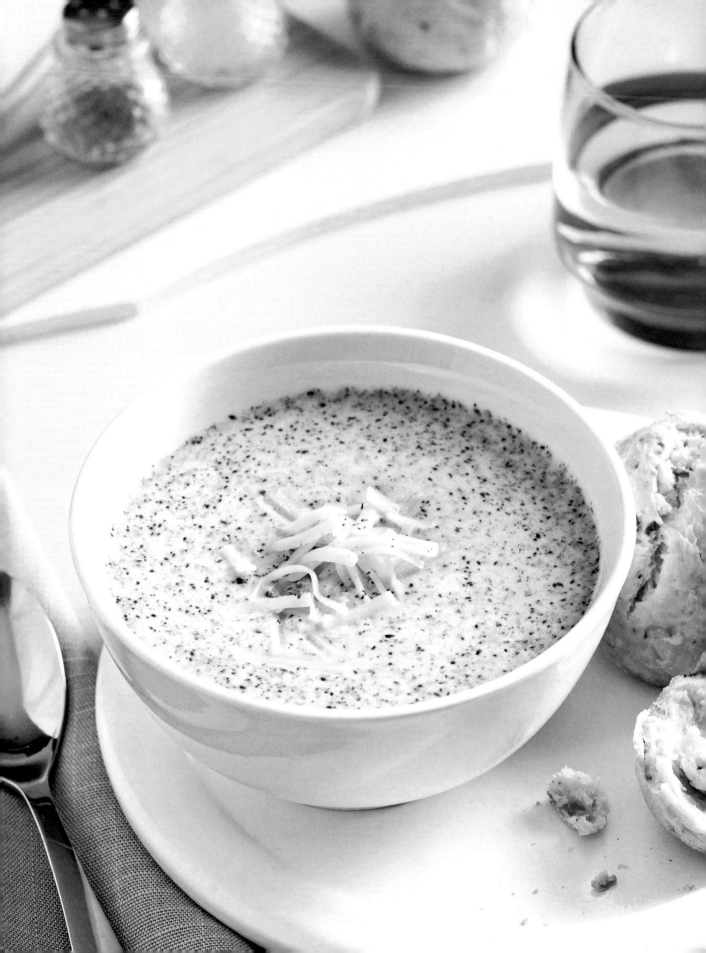

Tomato, Pepper and Beef Soup

Meal total
277
CALORIES

125 ml (½ cup) flour

30 ml (2 tbsp) paprika

10 ml (2 tsp) fresh thyme, chopped

5 ml (1 tsp) fresh rosemary, chopped

Salt and pepper to taste

450 g (1 lb) cubed beef stew meat, quartered

30 ml (2 tbsp) olive oil

2 carrots, diced

1 onion, diced

3 red peppers, diced

1 can (796 ml) diced tomatoes

1 bay leaf

10 ml (2 tsp) garlic, minced

2 litres (8 cups) beef stock

Prep time **25 minutes**

Cook time **35 minutes**

Serves **6**

PER SERVING	
Calories	277
Protein	21 g
Fat	11 g
Carbohydrates	23 g
Fibre	4 g
Iron	3 mg
Calcium	74 mg
Sodium	266 mg

1. Mix the flour with the paprika and herbs in a large bowl. Season with salt and pepper.

2. Add the beef cubes and stir to coat them in flour. Shake the cubes to remove excess flour and place them on a plate.

3. Heat the oil in a pot over medium heat. Brown the beef cubes.

4. Add the carrots and onion. Cook for 2 to 3 minutes.

5. Add the rest of the ingredients. Cover and let simmer over low heat for 35 to 40 minutes.

Did you know?

How to choose stock

Don't have time to make your own stock? Try a store bought version! To choose the right one, you should check the nutrition facts table first. A good stock contains less than 480 mg of sodium per 250 ml (1 cup). Be careful—just because a stock is labelled "low sodium" doesn't mean it actually is. And keep in mind that organic stocks are often an excellent choice!

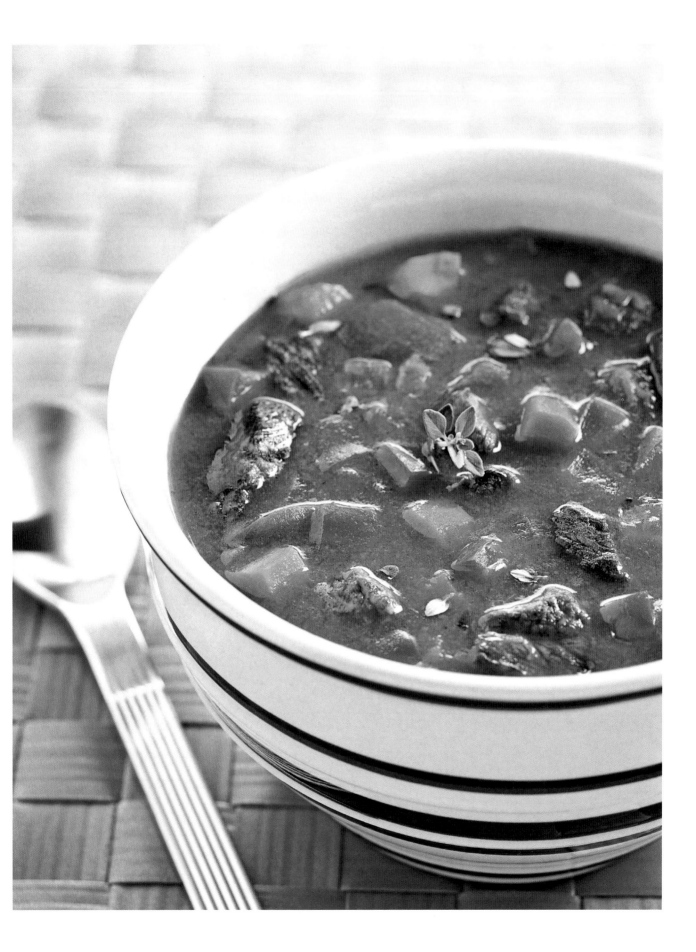

Tender Poultry

Use it in salads, stir-fries or sandwiches. Prepare it with Italian, Greek or Asian flavours. Any way you slice it, poultry is easily one of our favourite dishes! For gourmets on a diet, here are 13 poultry-based recipes that are as lean as they are delicious!

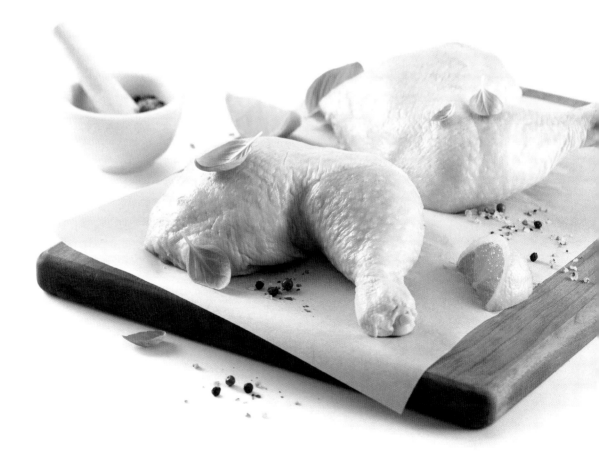

Spinach and Cheese Stuffed Chicken

Meal total
336
CALORIES

5 ml (1 tsp) canola oil

1 whole garlic clove, peeled

500 ml (2 cups) spinach, stems removed

450 g (1 lb) skinless chicken breasts

60 g fontina or mozzarella, sliced

30 ml (2 tbsp) sun-dried tomatoes, chopped

2.5 ml (½ tsp) salt

Freshly ground pepper, to taste

For the sauce:

160 ml (⅔ cup) plain Greek yogourt (0%)

10 ml (2 tsp) basil pesto

5 ml (1 tsp) honey

Prep time **30 minutes**

Cook time **20 minutes**

Serves **4**

PER SERVING	
Calories	250
Protein	34 g
Fat	10 g
Carbohydrates	5 g
Fibre	1 g
Iron	1 mg
Calcium	173 mg
Sodium	492 mg

1. Heat the oil in a frying pan over medium heat. Brown the garlic clove for 30 seconds. Remove the clove and throw it out.

2. Add the spinach to the pan and cook for a few seconds. Set aside on a plate and pat the spinach dry with paper towels.

3. Slice the chicken breasts in half horizontally, without cutting all the way through. Open like a book. Place the cheese, spinach and sun-dried tomatoes on one half of each breast. Season with salt and pepper.

4. Fold the other half of the breast over the filling and roll them up. Wrap the stuffed breasts in a large piece of plastic wrap and seal it completely.

5. Place the rolls in a large pot of boiling water. Lower the heat and poach for 20 minutes, until a thermometer inserted into the centre of a roll reads 74°C (165°F). Remove the rolls from the water and let cool before removing the plastic wrap.

6. Mix the sauce ingredients in a bowl.

7. Slice the chicken rolls and top with the sauce.

Try it with...

Arugula Walnut Salad
Per serving: 86 calories
Mix 750 ml (3 cups) arugula with 45 ml (3 tbsp) coarsely chopped walnuts. In a small bowl, mix 20 ml (4 tsp) olive oil with 20 ml (4 tsp) lemon juice. Pour onto the salad and toss. Season with salt and pepper.

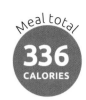

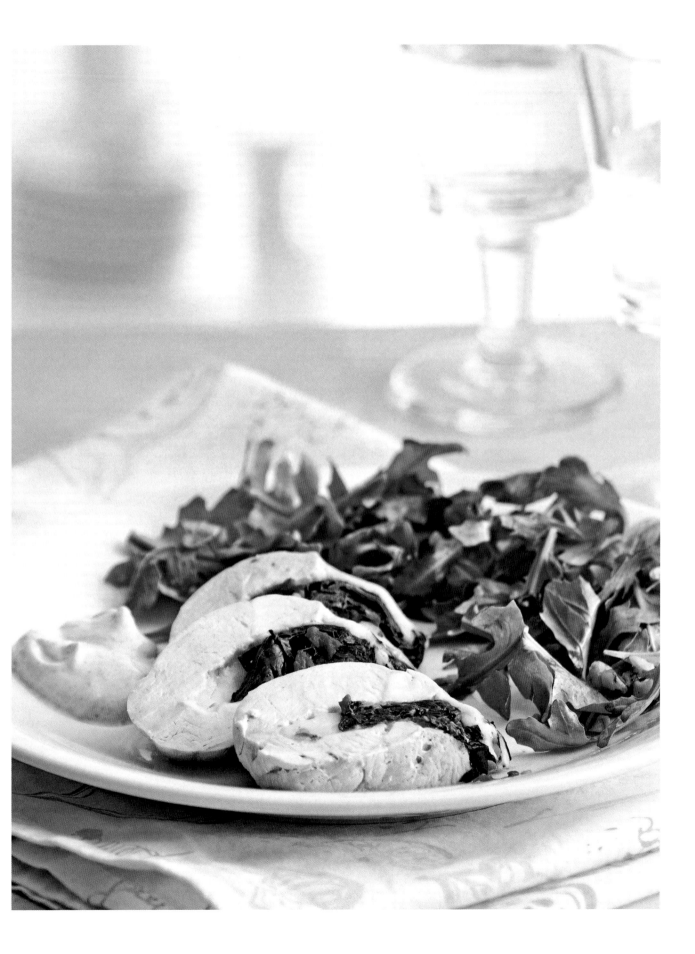

Greek Chicken Pita Pockets

Meal total
360
CALORIES

2 thick whole wheat pita pockets, cut in half

For the sauce:

375 ml (1 ½ cups) plain Greek yogourt (0%)

30 ml (2 tbsp) lemon juice

30 ml (2 tbsp) fresh cilantro, chopped

5 ml (1 tsp) cumin

5 ml (1 tsp) sambal oelek

1 garlic clove, minced

Salt to taste

For the chicken:

15 ml (1 tbsp) lemon juice

30 ml (2 tbsp) olive oil

Salt to taste

450 g (1 lb) chicken thighs, boneless and skinless

For the filling:

250 ml (1 cup) green cabbage, chopped

250 ml (1 cup) red cabbage, chopped

250 ml (1 cup) cucumbers, shredded

125 ml (½ cup) tomatoes, diced

Prep time **30 minutes**

Cook time **15 minutes**

Serves **4**

PER SERVING	
Calories	360
Protein	36 g
Fat	13 g
Carbohydrates	27 g
Fibre	5 g
Iron	3 mg
Calcium	193 mg
Sodium	357 mg

1. Mix all the sauce ingredients in a small bowl. Set aside.

2. Preheat the oven to 180°C (350°F).

3. In a larger bowl, mix the lemon juice with the oil and salt. Add the chicken and let marinate until the oven reaches the cooking temperature.

4. Place the chicken on a baking sheet lined with parchment paper. Bake for 15 to 20 minutes. Remove the baking sheet from the oven and let cool. Cut the chicken into strips.

5. Warm the pita pockets in the microwave for a few seconds and then fill them with the chicken, vegetables and sauce.

Try it because...

This sandwich is light but filling!
You might think that a sandwich stuffed so amply would hover around the 500 calorie mark—think again! Greek yogourt with 0% fat content is an excellent mayonnaise substitute, and chicken thighs are also low in fat. The whole wheat pita bread ties this sandwich together with a healthy dose of fiber, and it adds a nice texture, too.

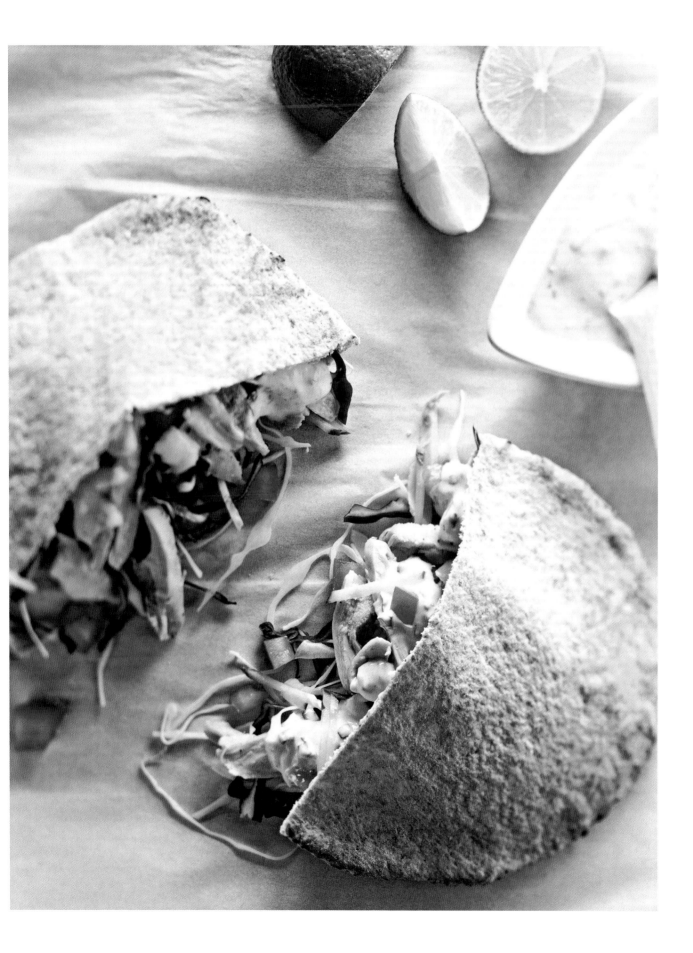

Pineapple Chicken Stir-Fry

Meal total
322
CALORIES

45 ml (3 tbsp) pineapple juice

15 ml (1 tbsp) canola oil

4 skinless chicken breasts,
cut into pieces

¼ pineapple, cut into pieces

1 red pepper, chopped

125 ml (½ cup) sweet
and sour stir-fry sauce

60 ml (¼ cup) water

15 ml (1 tbsp) lime zest

Salt and pepper to taste

2 green onions, chopped

Prep time **25 minutes**

Cook time **6 minutes**

Serves **4**

PER SERVING	
Calories	322
Protein	42 g
Fat	9 g
Carbohydrates	17 g
Fibre	2 g
Iron	1 mg
Calcium	26 mg
Sodium	252 mg

1. Heat the oil in a frying pan over medium heat. Sear the chicken for 2 minutes on each side.

2. Add the pineapple and pepper pieces. Cook for 2 to 3 minutes.

3. Add the sweet and sour sauce, water and lime zest. Season with salt and pepper. Bring to a boil.

4. Sprinkle each serving with green onions before serving.

Did you know?

It's a complete meal!

Convenient and easy to prepare, this stir-fry is a nutritious meal because it's made up of a protein source (chicken) and vegetables. And the lightly sweet taste comes from the pineapple, which is low in calories (41 calories for 125 ml—½ cup). The same serving size of pineapple also provides manganese, an element that is essential for bone formation, as well as nearly 13% of your daily vitamin C needs. Plus, this recipe only contains 11% of our recommended daily salt intake, which is reasonable. For a version with even less sodium, dilute two thirds of the sweet and sour sauce with about 45 ml (3 tbsp) of pineapple juice.

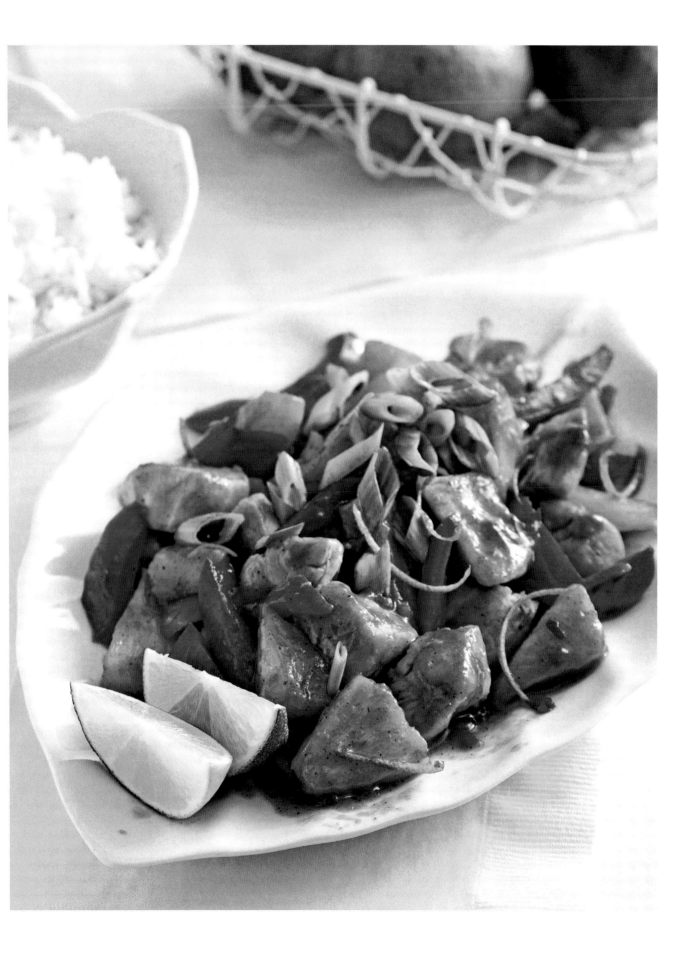

Chicken With Mushroom Sauce

Meal total
358
CALORIES

30 ml (2 tbsp) olive oil

680 g (1 ½ lb) chicken, cut into strips

125 ml (½ cup) dry white wine

250 ml (1 cup) veal stock

125 ml (½ cup) plain soy milk

1 package mushrooms, chopped

Prep time **15 minutes**

Cook time **8 minutes**

Serves **4**

PER SERVING	
Calories	305
Protein	46 g
Fat	9 g
Carbohydrates	3 g
Fibre	1 g
Iron	1 mg
Calcium	53 mg
Sodium	152 mg

1. Heat the oil in a frying pan over medium heat. Brown the chicken strips for 1 minute on each side. Transfer the meat to a plate and throw out the grease.

2. In the same pan, mix the wine with the veal stock and soy milk. Heat over medium heat until reduced by a quarter.

3. Put the chicken strips back into the pan and add the mushrooms. Cook for 8 to 10 minutes, until the chicken is cooked through.

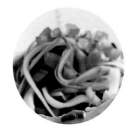

Try it with...

Zucchini and Squash Julienne
Per serving: 53 calories
Using a julienne cutter or peeler, slice 1 green zucchini and 1 yellow squash into thin julienne strips. Dice 1 tomato. Place the ingredients in a salad bowl and mix with 15 ml (1 tbsp) olive oil and 10 ml (2 tsp) cider vinegar. Season with salt and pepper.

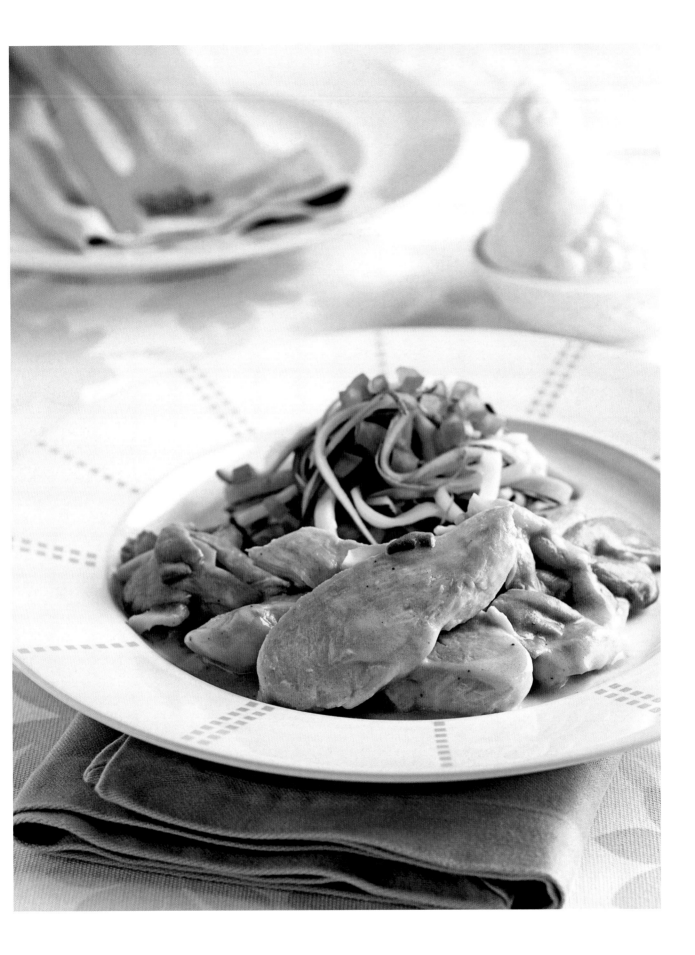

Turkey Puttanesca

450 g (1 lb) turkey cutlets, about 1 cm (½ in) thick

Salt and pepper to taste

10 ml (2 tsp) olive oil

2 garlic cloves, crushed

10 ml (2 tsp) anchovy paste or 2 anchovy fillets, finely chopped

60 ml (¼ cup) pitted black olives, cut in half

60 ml (¼ cup) capers, chopped

1 can (796 ml) diced tomatoes

80 ml (⅓ cup) water

A few stems parsley, chopped

Prep time **15 minutes**

Cook time **17 minutes**

Serves **4**

PER SERVING	
Calories	282
Protein	31 g
Fat	5 g
Carbohydrates	16 g
Fibre	4 g
Iron	4 mg
Calcium	94 mg
Sodium	781 mg

1. Season the cutlets with salt and pepper.

2. Heat the oil in a non-stick pan over medium heat. Brown the cutlets for about 2 minutes on each side. Remove and set aside on a plate.

3. In the same pan, add the garlic and anchovy. Cook for 1 minute.

4. Add the olives, capers and tomatoes. Cook over medium heat for about 5 more minutes, until the sauce has slightly thickened.

5. Adjust the seasoning as needed and add the water. Stir and then put the cutlets into the sauce. Cook for another 7 minutes, until the turkey shreds easily with a fork.

6. Garnish each serving with parsley before serving.

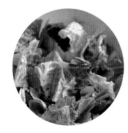

Try it with...

Green Salad
Per serving: 86 calories
In a salad bowl, whisk together 30 ml (2 tbsp) olive oil with 15 ml (1 tbsp) sherry vinegar and 10 ml (2 tsp) honey. Add 750 ml (3 cups) shredded romaine lettuce and 1 shredded carrot. Season with salt and pepper.

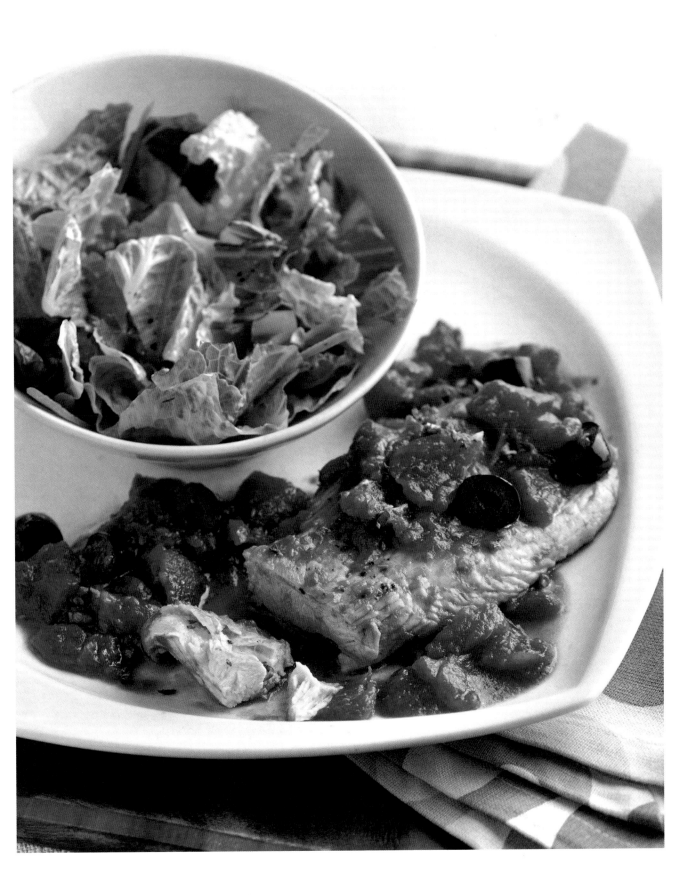

Asian Chicken Stir-Fry

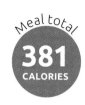

Meal total
381
CALORIES

1 carrot

1 red pepper

1 red onion

½ broccoli

15 ml (1 tbsp) canola oil

100 g snow peas

3 skinless chicken breasts, chopped

10 ml (2 tsp) garlic, minced

250 ml (1 cup) orange and ginger stir-fry sauce

60 ml (¼ cup) peanuts

2 green onions, chopped (optional)

Prep time **25 minutes**

Cook time **8 minutes**

Serves **4**

PER SERVING	
Calories	381
Protein	33 g
Fat	12 g
Carbohydrates	36 g
Fibre	3 g
Iron	5 mg
Calcium	33 mg
Sodium	566 mg

1. Slice the carrot, pepper and onion. Cut the broccoli into small florets.

2. Heat the oil in a frying pan or wok over medium heat. Sear the sliced vegetables, broccoli and snow peas for 3 to 4 minutes. Transfer to a plate and set aside.

3. In the same pan, cook the chicken for 2 minutes on each side, working in small batches. Add the garlic and sauce. Heat for 1 to 2 minutes.

4. Sprinkle each serving with peanuts and green onions before serving.

It's easy!

Perfect your stir-fry

1. Stir-fry is meant to be cooked quickly, so prepare all the ingredients before you turn on the stove.
2. Choose an oil with a neutral taste and a high smoke point, like peanut, canola or sunflower oil.
3. Always cook meat, poultry or seafood separately from the vegetables.
4. It's a good idea to blanch less tender vegetables, like cauliflower and broccoli, beforehand. Cook them for 2 to 3 minutes in a pot of boiling salted water.

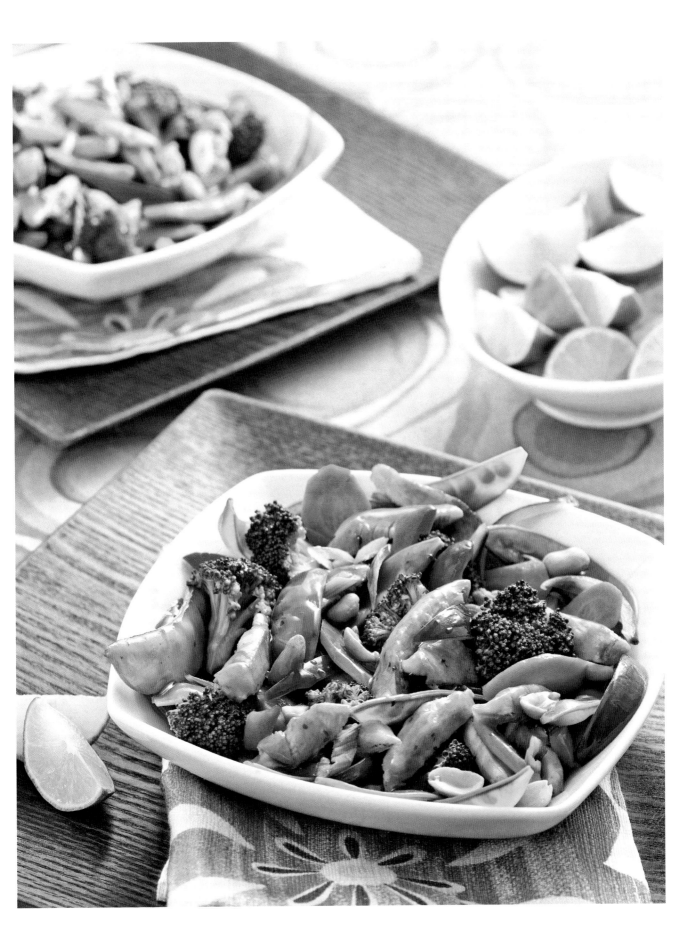

Lemon Honey Chicken

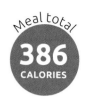

15 ml (1 tbsp) olive oil

4 skinless chicken breasts

For the vinaigrette:

45 ml (3 tbsp) olive oil

45 ml (3 tbsp) lemon juice

45 ml (3 tbsp) fresh chives, chopped

30 ml (2 tbsp) honey

15 ml (1 tbsp) lemon zest

5 ml (1 tsp) fresh thyme, chopped

Salt and pepper to taste

For the salad:

1 head curly leaf lettuce

½ red onion

18 cherry tomatoes, various colours

Prep time **25 minutes**

Cook time **12 minutes**

Serves **4**

PER SERVING	
Calories	386
Protein	41 g
Fat	17 g
Carbohydrates	18 g
Fibre	2 g
Iron	2 mg
Calcium	61 mg
Sodium	177 mg

1. Whisk together the vinaigrette ingredients in a bowl. Pour half of the vinaigrette into a salad bowl and put it in the refrigerator (it will be used to dress the salad). Set aside the rest of the vinaigrette for cooking.

2. Preheat the oven to 205°C (400°F).

3. Heat the olive oil in an ovenproof skillet over medium heat. Brown the chicken breasts for 1 to 2 minutes on each side. Transfer the breasts to a plate.

4. Pour the cooking vinaigrette into the skillet and bring to a boil, scraping the bottom of the skillet with a wooden spoon. Put the breasts back into the skillet, turning them so that they are fully coated in the sauce.

5. Bake for 10 to 12 minutes, until the chicken is no longer pink in the centre.

6. While the chicken is cooking, prepare the salad. Remove the stems from the lettuce. Chop the onion and cut the cherry tomatoes in half. Place the vegetables in the salad bowl containing the vinaigrette. Toss. Serve with the sliced chicken breasts.

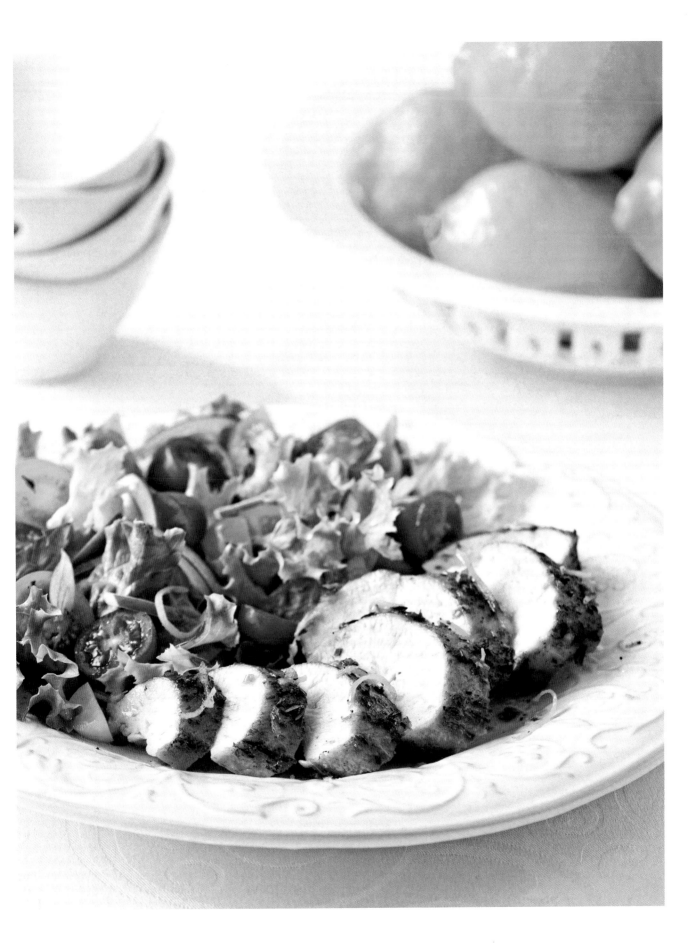

Sesame Chicken Stir-Fry

180 ml (¾ cup) basmati rice

For the marinade:

60 ml (¼ cup) hoisin sauce

30 ml (2 tbsp) soy sauce (low-sodium)

15 ml (1 tbsp) rice vinegar

15 ml (1 tbsp) lime juice

1.25 ml (¼ tsp) pepper flakes

1 garlic clove, minced

For the stir-fry:

15 ml (1 tbsp) canola oil

450 g (1 lb) chicken breasts, cut into strips

7.5 ml (½ tbsp) toasted sesame oil

500 ml (2 cups) snow peas

125 ml (½ cup) water

30 ml (2 tbsp) sesame seeds

Cilantro leaves, chopped

Prep time **20 minutes**

Cook time **10 minutes**

Serves **4**

PER SERVING	
Calories	400
Protein	31 g
Fat	12 g
Carbohydrates	40 g
Fibre	2 g
Iron	2 mg
Calcium	58 mg
Sodium	611 mg

1. Cook the rice according to the instructions on the packaging.

2. Mix the marinade ingredients in a bowl. Set aside.

3. Heat the canola oil in a frying pan or a wok over medium heat. Cook the chicken over high heat for 2 minutes on each side, until it is cooked through and lightly browned. Remove from the pan and set aside.

4. In the same pan, add the sesame oil, snow peas, marinade and water. Cook over medium heat for 3 minutes.

5. Put the chicken back into the pan and add the sesame seeds. Cook for a few more minutes, stirring so that the ingredients are fully coated in the marinade.

6. Distribute the rice onto plates. Top with the stir-fry and sprinkle with cilantro.

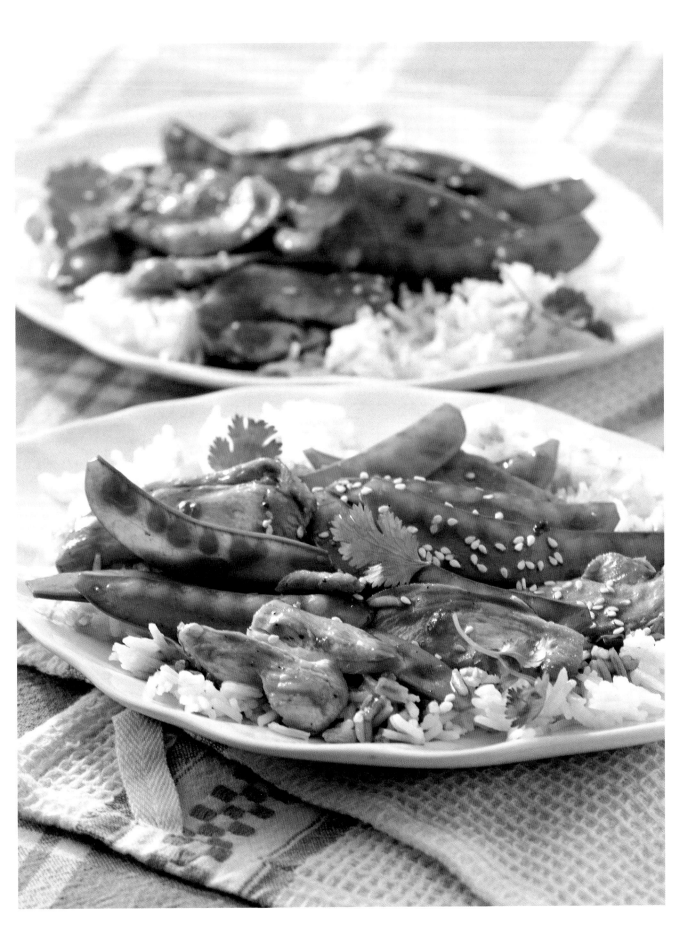

Chicken Tortilla Cups

Meal total
381
CALORIES

4 small whole wheat tortillas

500 ml (2 cups) milk

80 ml (⅓ cup) unbleached, all-purpose flour

15 ml (1 tbsp) Dijon mustard

Salt and pepper to taste

25 asparagus spears, cut into pieces

15 ml (1 tbsp) olive oil

500 ml (2 cups) fresh mushrooms, sliced

500 ml (2 cups) cooked chicken, cut into pieces

Prep time **30 minutes**

Cook time **15 minutes**

Serves **4**

PER SERVING	
Calories	381
Protein	35 g
Fat	12 g
Carbohydrates	34 g
Fibre	5 g
Iron	4 mg
Calcium	192 mg
Sodium	487 mg

1. Preheat the oven to 190°C (375°F).

2. Place the tortillas into the cups of a muffin tin and form them into little bowls (if needed, microwave the tortillas for a few seconds to soften them). Brown in the oven for 7 minutes. Remove from the oven and let cool.

3. Pour the milk into a pot. Use a sifter to sprinkle the flour into the milk, whisking until smooth. Bring to a boil and simmer until the mixture thickens, whisking constantly. Remove from heat. Add the mustard. Season with salt and pepper.

4. Cook the asparagus for 3 minutes in a large pot of boiling, salted water. Submerge in ice water and then drain.

5. Heat the oil over medium-high heat in a non-stick pan. Brown the mushrooms for 4 minutes. Add the chicken and asparagus. Stir and then transfer to the béchamel sauce. Mix well and adjust the seasoning as needed.

6. Spoon the filling into the tortilla bowls.

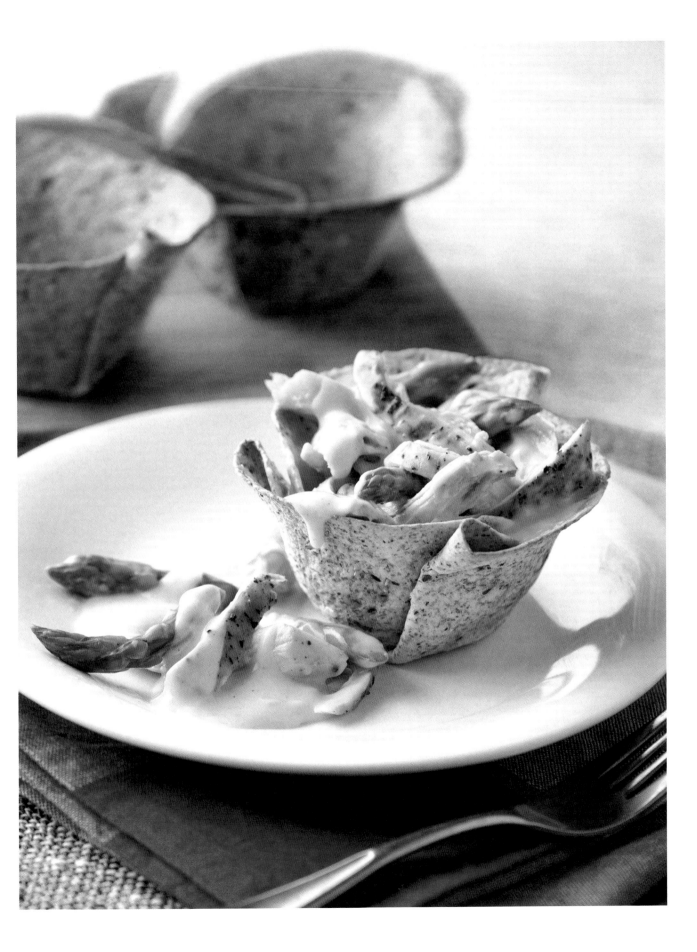

Pepper Stuffed Chicken Breasts

Meal total
381
CALORIES

4 skinless chicken breasts

1 red or yellow pepper, thinly sliced

50 g (1 ¾ oz) light cheddar, cut into sticks

8 green beans, cut in half

4 sprigs thyme

Salt and pepper to taste

15 ml (1 tbsp) olive oil

80 ml (⅓ cup) white wine

60 ml (¼ cup) shallots, chopped

Prep time **20 minutes**

Cook time **18 minutes**

Serves **4**

PER SERVING	
Calories	286
Protein	38 g
Fat	10 g
Carbohydrates	6 g
Fibre	1 g
Iron	1 mg
Calcium	144 mg
Sodium	163 mg

1. Preheat the oven to 190°C (375°F).

2. Slice the chicken breasts in half horizontally, without cutting all the way through.

3. Stuff the breasts with pepper, cheddar, green beans and the sprigs of thyme. Use toothpicks to keep the breasts closed. Season with salt and pepper.

4. Heat the oil in an ovenproof skillet over medium heat. Brown the breasts for 1 minute on each side.

5. Add the white wine and shallots.

6. Cover and bake for 16 to 18 minutes, until the chicken is no longer pink in the centre.

Try it with...

Fresh Salad
Per serving: 95 calories
In a salad bowl, mix 15 ml (1 tbsp) olive oil with 30 ml (2 tbsp) orange juice, 30 ml (2 tbsp) fresh chives, chopped, and 30 ml (2 tbsp) pistachios, chopped. Season with salt and pepper. Add 8 cherry tomatoes, quartered, 2 mini cucumbers, thinly sliced, 1 fennel bulb, thinly sliced, and 500 ml (2 cups) spring mix lettuce. Toss.

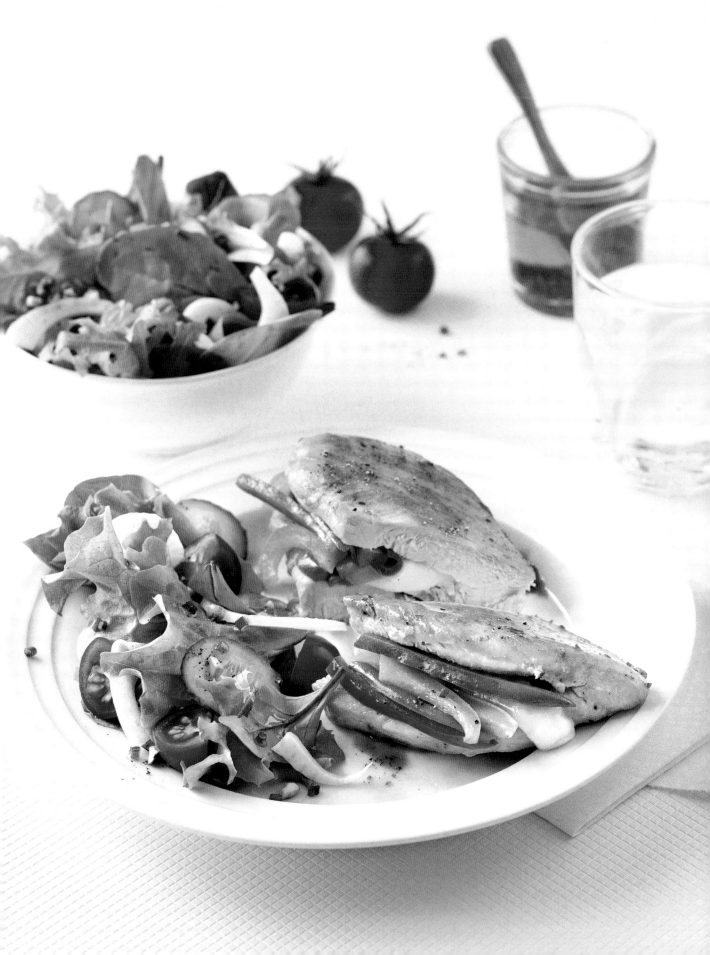

Sheet Pan Fajitas

80 ml (⅓ cup) plain Greek yogourt (0%)

10 ml (2 tsp) paprika

1 packet (24 g) fajita seasoning

45 ml (3 tbsp)
fresh cilantro, chopped

15 ml (1 tbsp) lime zest

3 skinless chicken breasts, cut into pieces

3 pepper halves, various colours, thinly sliced

1 onion, thinly sliced

2 tomatoes, cut into wedges

Pepper to taste

12 small tortillas

Prep time **20 minutes**

Cook time **15 minutes**

Serves **6**

PER SERVING	
Calories	384
Protein	35 g
Fat	8 g
Carbohydrates	40 g
Fibre	3 g
Iron	2 mg
Calcium	52 mg
Sodium	901 mg

1. Preheat the oven to 190°C (375°F).

2. In a bowl, mix the yogourt with the paprika, fajita seasoning, cilantro, lime zest and pieces of chicken.

3. Spread the prepared chicken onto a baking sheet lined with parchment paper. Add the peppers, onion and tomatoes. Season with pepper and stir.

4. Bake for 15 to 18 minutes, until the chicken is no longer pink in the centre.

5. Top the tortillas with the chicken and vegetables and then roll them up tightly.

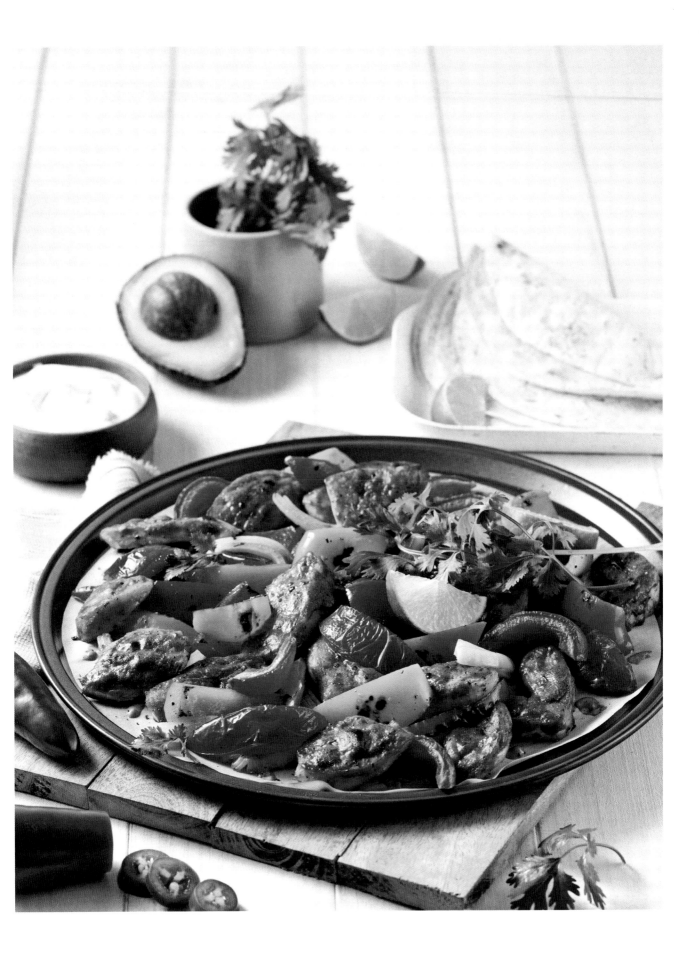

Indian Butter Chicken

Meal total 373 CALORIES

For the chicken:

5 ml (1 tsp) turmeric

1.25 ml (¼ tsp) ground cardamom

1.25 ml (¼ tsp) ground cloves

1.25 ml (¼ tsp) cinnamon

15 ml (1 tbsp) garam masala

675 g (about 1 ½ lb) chicken, cut into cubes

125 ml (½ cup) plain yogourt (0%)

1 can (540 ml) diced tomatoes

60 ml (¼ cup) almond flour

80 ml (⅓ cup) chicken stock

1 Thai chili pepper

30 ml (2 tbsp) tomato paste

15 ml (1 tbsp) canola oil

1 onion, chopped

15 ml (1 tbsp) garlic, minced

15 ml (1 tbsp) ginger, minced

Cilantro leaves to taste (optional)

For the vegetables:

15 ml (1 tbsp) canola oil

2 carrots, cut into rounds

1 red pepper, cut into cubes

1 zucchini, chopped

Salt and pepper to taste

Prep time **25 minutes**

Marination **30 minutes**

Cook time **30 minutes**

Serves **6**

PER SERVING	
Calories	250
Protein	30 g
Fat	7 g
Carbohydrates	16 g
Fibre	3 g
Iron	2 mg
Calcium	108 mg
Sodium	261 mg

1. Mix the spices in a large bowl. Add the chicken and stir to coat it with spices. Cover with plastic wrap and let marinate for 30 minutes in the refrigerator.

2. In a blender, add the yogourt, diced tomatoes, almond flour, chicken stock, chili pepper and tomato paste and blend until smooth and evenly mixed.

3. Heat the canola oil in a frying pan over medium heat. Brown the chicken cubes for 2 to 3 minutes.

4. Add the onion, garlic and ginger. Cook for 1 minute. Stir in the yogourt mixture. Bring to a boil, and then cover and cook for 25 to 30 minutes over low heat.

5. Heat the oil in another frying pan over medium heat. Cook the carrots for 2 to 3 minutes. Add the pepper and cook for another 2 minutes. Add the zucchini and cook for 1 minute. Season with salt and pepper. Serve with the chicken.

6. If desired, sprinkle each serving with cilantro leaves.

Try it with...

Kaffir Lime-Flavoured Rice
Per serving: 123 calories
In a pot, place 250 ml (1 cup) rice, 2 kaffir lime leaves and 500 ml (2 cups) chicken stock. Season with salt and pepper. Bring to a boil, and then cover and cook for 18 to 20 minutes over medium-low heat.

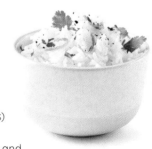

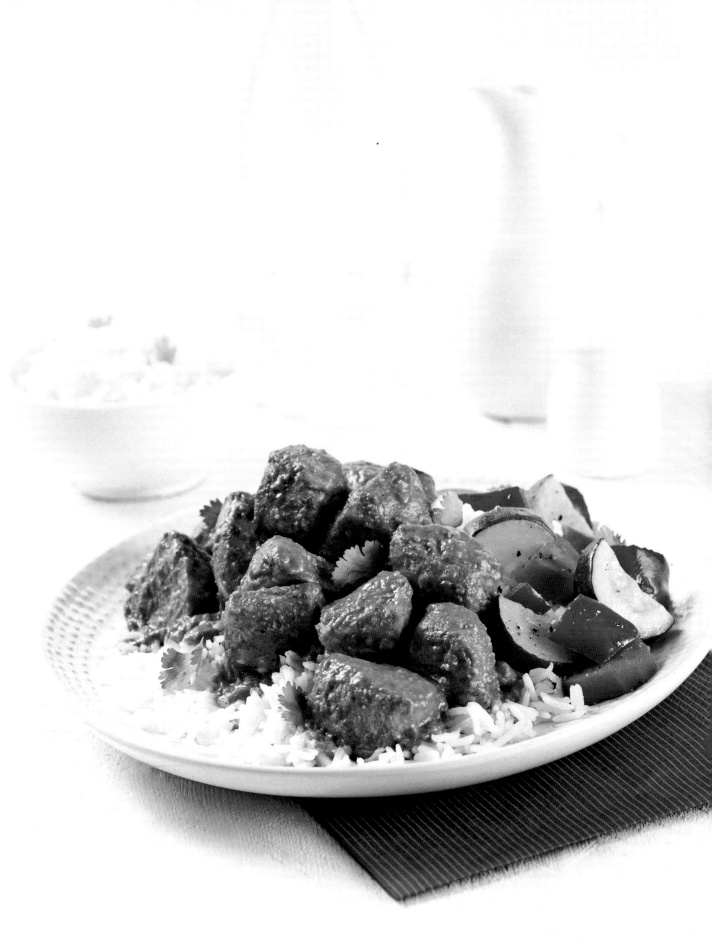

Crispy Spice-Rubbed Chicken Legs

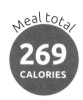

Meal total

269 CALORIES

4 skinless chicken legs

15 ml (1 tbsp) olive oil

For the spice rub:

15 ml (1 tbsp) paprika

15 ml (1 tbsp) lemon zest

15 ml (1 tbsp) brown sugar

10 ml (2 tsp) cumin

5 ml (1 tsp) garlic powder

Salt and pepper to taste

For the vegetables:

20 green beans

20 yellow beans

2 large carrots, cut into pieces

30 ml (2 tbsp) water

15 ml (1 tbsp) olive oil

Salt and pepper to taste

1 sprig of thyme

Prep time **15 minutes**

Cook time **30 minutes**

Serves **4**

PER SERVING	
Calories	269
Protein	27 g
Fat	13 g
Carbohydrates	12 g
Fibre	3 g
Iron	3 mg
Calcium	66 mg
Sodium	157 mg

1. Preheat the oven to 220°C (425°F).

2. Mix all the spice rub ingredients in a deep plate.

3. Coat the chicken legs in the spice mix. Place the legs on a baking sheet lined with parchment paper and drizzle with oil.

4. Bake for 30 to 35 minutes.

5. Place the vegetables on a large piece of aluminum foil. Pour the water and olive oil over the vegetables. Season with salt and pepper. Place the sprig of thyme on the vegetables and then fold over the aluminum foil to form an airtight packet. Place onto a baking sheet and bake for 15 minutes, until the packet is puffed.

6. Serve the vegetables with the chicken.

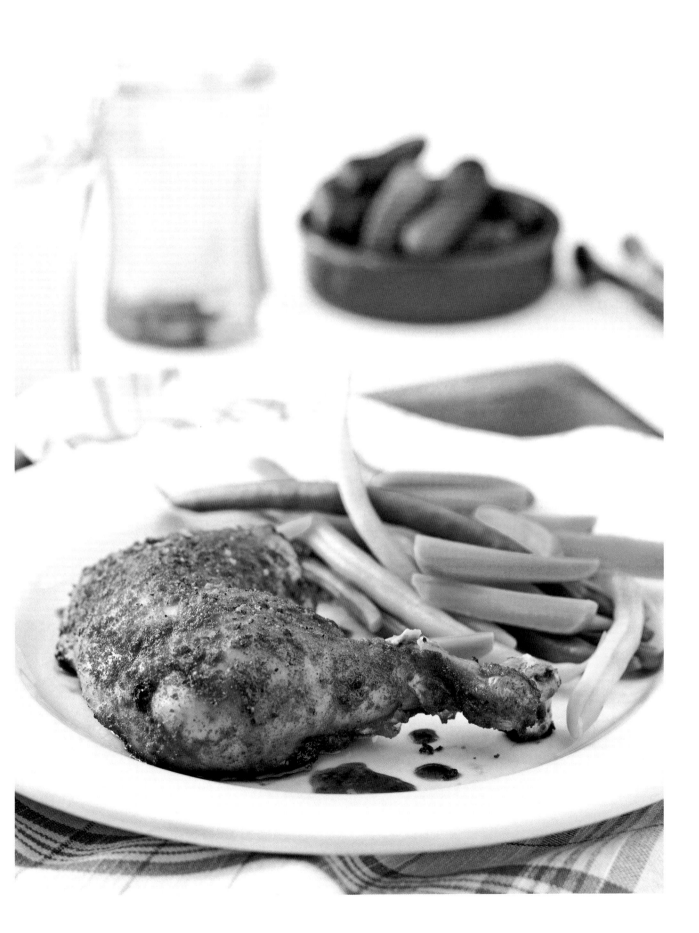

Seafood Delicacies

Seafood paella, honey mustard seared scallops, tuna quesadillas... the sea is overflowing with low-calorie delicacies! Want to find out more? Check out our delectable ideas in the next section!

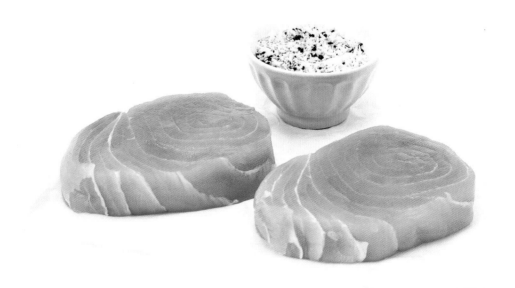

Seafood Paella

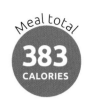

Meal total
383
CALORIES

5 ml (1 tsp) saffron

625 ml (2 ½ cups) vegetable stock

30 ml (2 tbsp) olive oil

350 g (about ¾ lb) frozen diced vegetable mix, thawed and drained

15 ml (1 tbsp) garlic, minced

310 ml (1 ¼ cups) long grain white rice

1 bag (340 g) frozen mixed shrimp and scallops, thawed and drained

4 Italian tomatoes, diced

45 ml (3 tbsp) fresh parsley, chopped

Prep time **15 minutes**

Cook time **16 minutes**

Serves **4**

PER SERVING	
Calories	383
Protein	18 g
Fat	8 g
Carbohydrates	61 g
Fibre	3 g
Iron	1 mg
Calcium	76 mg
Sodium	927 mg

1. Infuse the saffron in the heated vegetable stock.

2. Heat the oil in a pot over medium heat. Sear the vegetables and garlic for 1 to 2 minutes.

3. Add the rice. Pour in the stock and bring to a boil over medium heat. Cover and cook for 12 to 15 minutes.

4. Add the seafood, tomatoes and parsley. Cook for another 3 to 5 minutes.

Also try it...

On the barbecue
Follow these steps to cook this paella on the barbecue. Infuse the saffron in the heated vegetable stock. Heat a paella pan or a large, heavy-bottomed pot on the grill over medium-high heat. Sear the vegetables and garlic for 1 to 2 minutes in the oil. Add the rice. Pour in the stock and bring to a boil. Close the lid and cook for 12 to 15 minutes. Add the seafood, tomatoes, and parsley. Stir. Close the lid and cook for another 3 to 5 minutes.

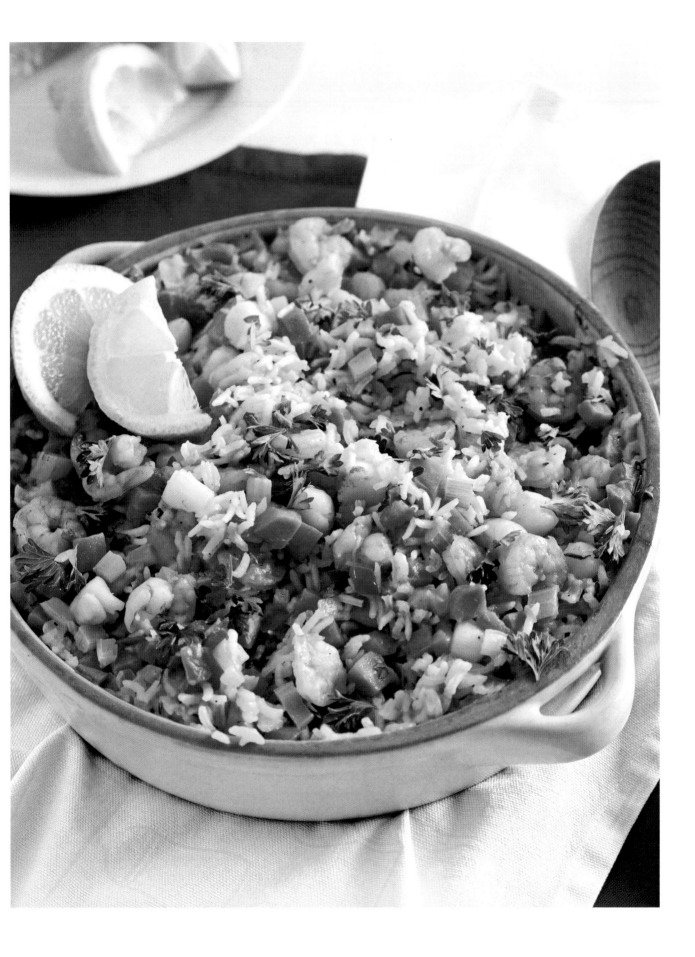

Sole Fillets With Avocado and Tomato

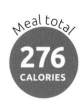

Meal total
276
CALORIES

1 avocado

3 tomatoes

30 ml (2 tbsp) olive oil

30 ml (2 tbsp) lemon juice

5 ml (1 tsp) fresh chives, chopped

A few sprigs dill

3 green onions, chopped

125 ml (½ cup) vegetable stock

8 sole fillets, 80 g (about ⅕ lb) each

Prep time **20 minutes**

Cook time **8 minutes**

Serves **4**

PER SERVING	
Calories	276
Protein	22 g
Fat	18 g
Carbohydrates	9 g
Fibre	5 g
Iron	1 mg
Calcium	59 mg
Sodium	563 mg

1. Dice the avocado and tomatoes and place in a bowl. Add the oil, lemon juice, chives, dill and green onions. Stir.

2. Heat the stock in a large frying pan over medium heat. Roll up the sole fillets and place them in the pan. Cover and cook for 6 to 8 minutes.

3. Add the avocado mix to the pan. Cover and cook for 2 to 3 minutes.

Did you know?

Poaching has many benefits

There are many ways to cook fish. It can be baked, fried or grilled, but there's another method that we tend to forget—poaching fish in stock. Not only is this technique easy to pull off, it also preserves the nutritional properties and tender texture of the fish without adding extra fat. You'll need to cook the fish for 8 to 10 minutes for every inch (2.5 cm) of thickness.

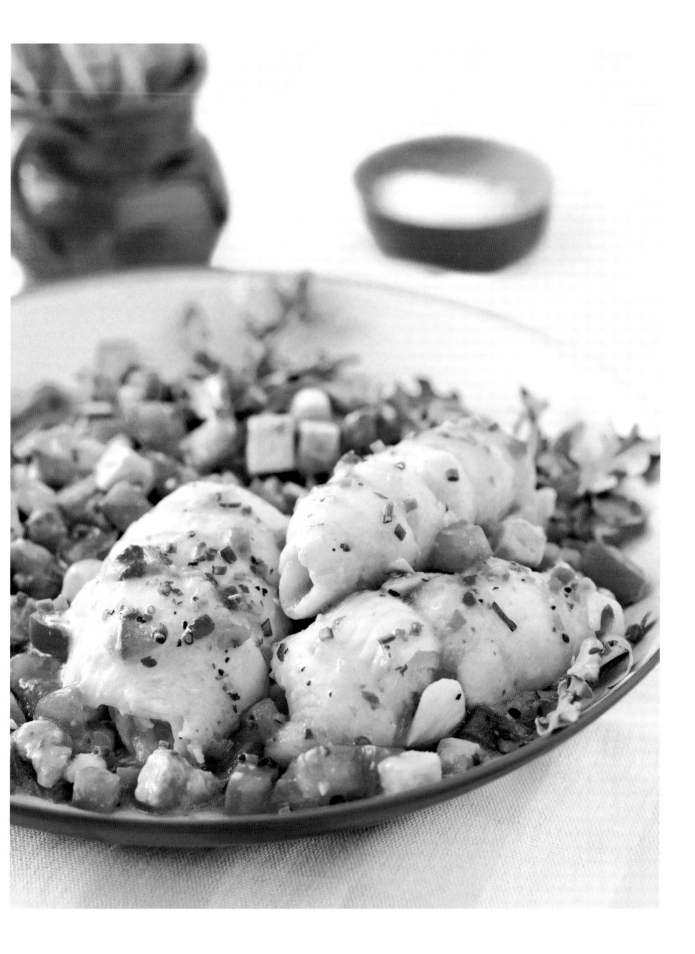

Honey Mustard Seared Scallops

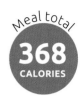

Meal total
368
CALORIES

20 snow peas

For the scallops:

15 ml (1 tbsp) olive oil

350 g (about ¾ lb) scallops (U/12 count)

20 ml (4 tsp) butter

60 ml (¼ cup) honey

30 ml (2 tbsp) lemon juice

45 ml (3 tbsp) whole-grain mustard

3 tomatoes, diced

15 ml (1 tbsp) lemon zest

For the rice:

180 ml (¾ cup) white rice

375 ml (1 ½ cups) chicken stock

30 ml (2 tbsp) fresh parsley, chopped

Prep time **15 minutes**

Cook time **15 minutes**

Serves **4**

PER SERVING	
Calories	368
Protein	16 g
Fat	9 g
Carbohydrates	57 g
Fibre	3 g
Iron	2 mg
Calcium	50 mg
Sodium	858 mg

1. In a pot, cook the rice in the chicken stock according to the instructions on the packaging.

2. Place a steamer basket in another pot. Add water to the bottom of the pot and place the snow peas in the steamer basket. Bring the water to a boil and cook the snow peas until tender.

3. Once the rice and snow peas are cooked, heat the oil in a frying pan over medium heat. Sear the scallops for 30 seconds on each side. Remove from the pan and set aside on a plate.

4. In the same pan, melt the butter over medium heat. Add the honey and heat for 1 to 2 minutes until the butter becomes amber in colour. Add the lemon juice, mustard, diced tomatoes and zest. Bring to a boil and reduce to low heat. Cook for 1 minute.

5. Put the scallops back in the pan. Heat for 1 minute.

6. Serve the scallops with the rice and snow peas. Sprinkle each serving with chopped parsley.

Did you know?

How to achieve tender scallops

When purchasing scallops, remember that they're categorized by count: the number corresponds to how many scallops you get per pound. The lower the number, the bigger the scallop, and vice versa. Scallops should be cooked very quickly. Otherwise, the meat becomes hard, dry and less tasty. After one or two minutes, scallops become opaque—it means they're done. In terms of health, scallops are a great choice because they have a very low fat content and are an excellent source of both protein and calcium.

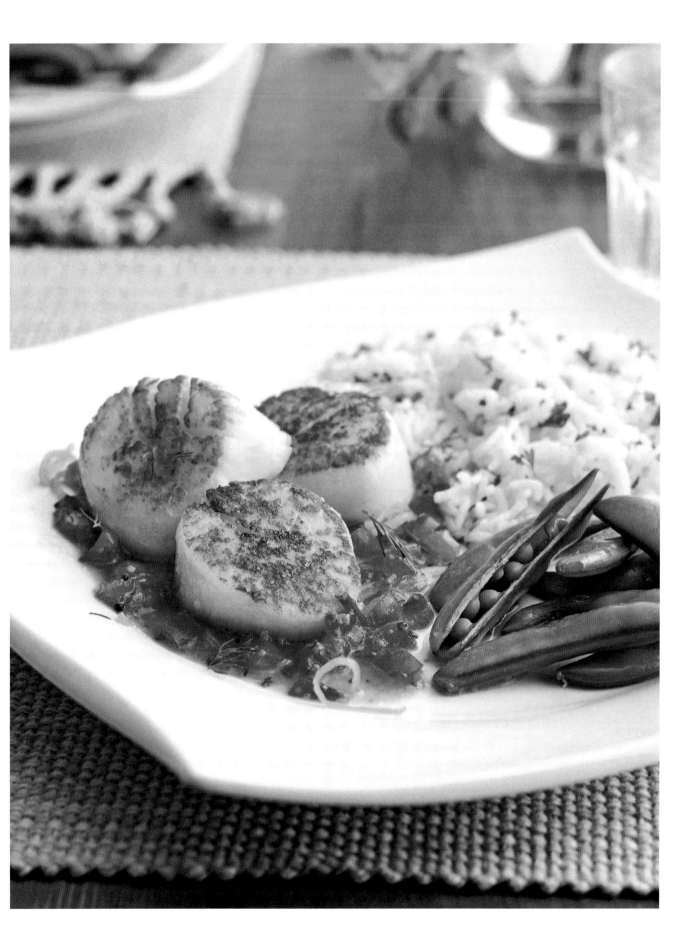

Shrimp and Scallops With Maple Vinaigrette

Meal total
225
CALORIES

15 ml (1 tbsp) olive oil

12 jumbo shrimp (16-20 count), raw and peeled

12 scallops (15-25 count)

2 green onions, chopped

1 bag (283 g) angel hair coleslaw

Salt and pepper to taste

80 ml (⅓ cup) maple vinaigrette

Prep time **20 minutes**

Cook time **4 minutes**

Serves **4**

PER SERVING	
Calories	225
Protein	20 g
Fat	11 g
Carbohydrates	12 g
Fibre	3 g
Iron	1 mg
Calcium	83 mg
Sodium	771 mg

1. Heat the olive oil in a frying pan over medium heat. Sear the shrimp and scallops for 1 to 2 minutes on each side. Remove from the pan and set aside on a plate.

2. In the same pan, cook the green onions and coleslaw for 1 to 2 minutes. Season with salt and pepper.

3. Add the seafood and maple vinaigrette. Cook for 1 minute.

Did you know?

What is angel hair coleslaw?
If you're a fan of fresh salads that can be tossed together in a flash, we've got good news! Most supermarkets sell ready-to-eat coleslaw mixes. The finely cut cabbage used in this recipe is high in fibre and vitamin C and looks like the aptly named "angel hair" pasta. Its delicate cut makes it an excellent choice for soaking up the flavour of the vinaigrette. To make it at home, thinly slice some cabbage leaves.

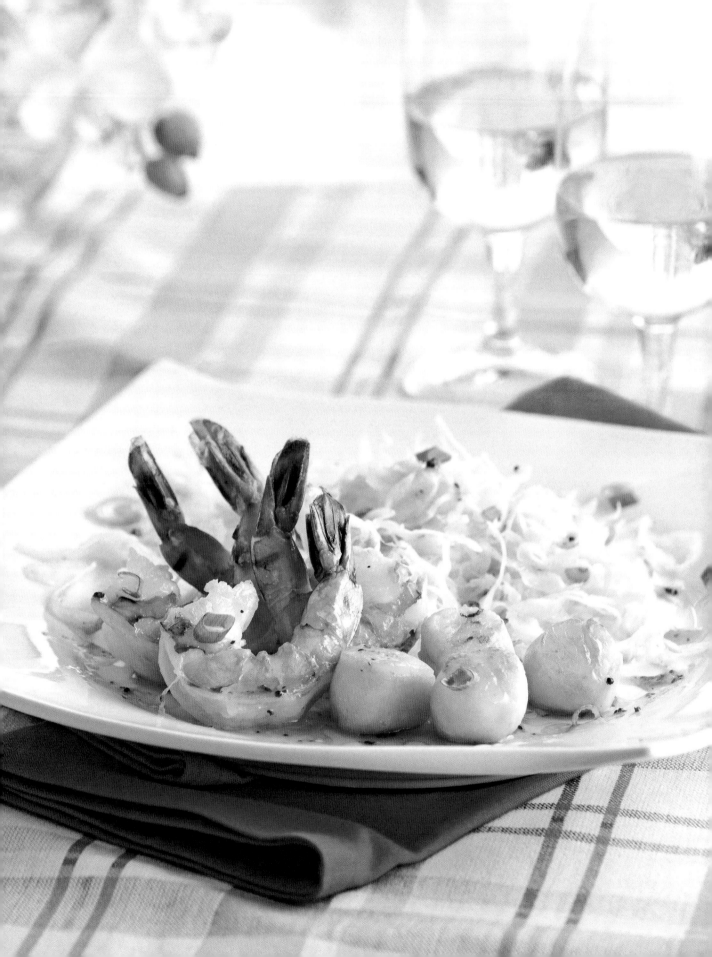

Meal total
388
CALORIES

Tuna Quesadillas

2 cans tuna, 120 g each, drained

180 ml (¾ cup) Tex-Mex shredded cheese

80 ml (⅓ cup) salsa

125 ml (½ cup) carrots, cut into thin julienne strips

125 ml (½ cup) zucchinis, cut into thin julienne strips

45 ml (3 tbsp) fresh cilantro, chopped

4 medium tortillas

15 ml (1 tbsp) olive oil

Prep time **15 minutes**

Cook time **6 minutes**

Serves **4**

PER SERVING	
Calories	298
Protein	25 g
Fat	13 g
Carbohydrates	21 g
Fibre	4 g
Iron	2 mg
Calcium	197 mg
Sodium	619 mg

1. In a bowl, mix the tuna with the cheese, salsa, julienne vegetables and cilantro.

2. Distribute the mixture onto half of each tortilla. Fold the tortillas over the filling.

3. Heat the oil in a frying pan over medium-low heat. Cook the tortillas for 3 minutes on each side.

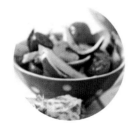

Try it with...

Garden Salad
Per serving: 90 calories
In a salad bowl, mix 30 ml (2 tbsp) olive oil with 5 ml (1 tsp) lemon juice. Season with salt and pepper. Chop ½ cucumber, ½ yellow pepper and ½ red onion. Add the vegetables to the salad bowl with 12 cherry tomatoes of various colours, cut in half. Toss.

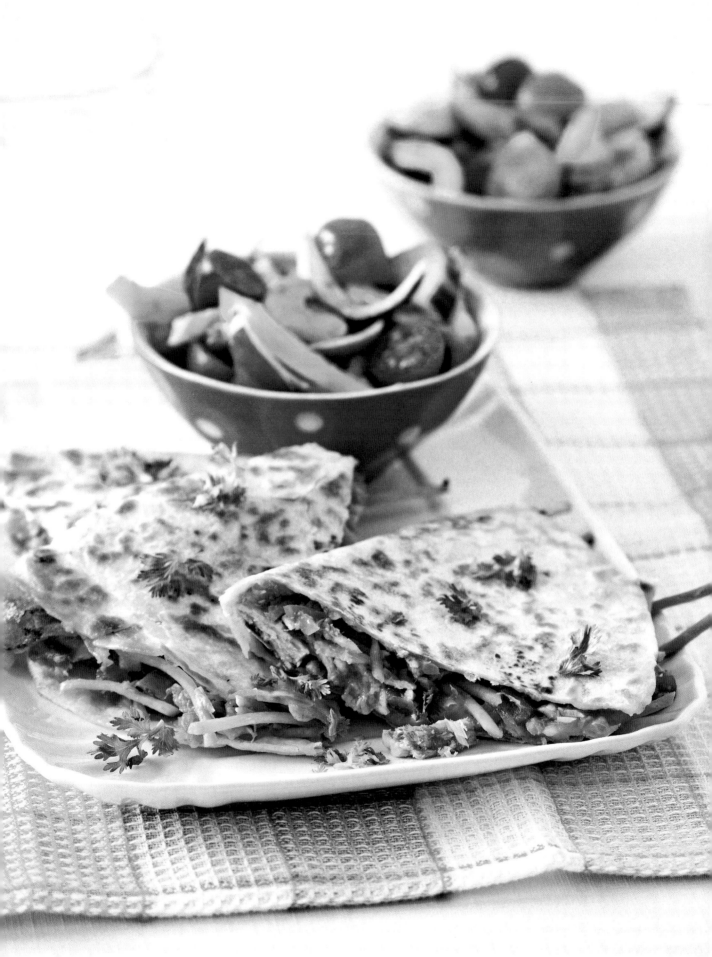

Salmon Fillets With Honey Orange Sauce

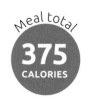

Meal total 375 CALORIES

4 salmon fillets, 180 g
(about ⅓ lb) each

For the sauce:

80 ml (⅓ cup) frozen orange
juice concentrate, thawed

30 ml (2 tbsp) honey

30 ml (2 tbsp) shallots,
chopped

15 ml (1 tbsp) ginger, minced

Salt and pepper to taste

Prep time **10 minutes**

Cook time **10 minutes**

Serves **4**

PER SERVING	
Calories	303
Protein	36 g
Fat	11 g
Carbohydrates	12 g
Fibre	0 g
Iron	2 mg
Calcium	27 mg
Sodium	81 mg

1. Preheat the oven to 205°C
(400°F).

2. Mix the sauce ingredients
in a bowl.

3. Place the salmon fillets in a
baking dish, skin side down. Pour
the sauce onto the fish.

4. Bake for 10 to 12 minutes, until
the meat flakes easily with a fork.

Try it with...

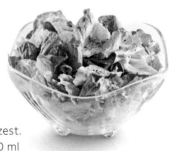

Mixed Green Salad
Per serving: 72 calories
In a salad bowl, whisk together 30 ml
(2 tbsp) olive oil with 15 ml (1 tbsp)
lemon juice and 15 ml (1 tbsp) lemon zest.
Season with salt and pepper. Add 750 ml
(3 cups) mixed greens and toss.

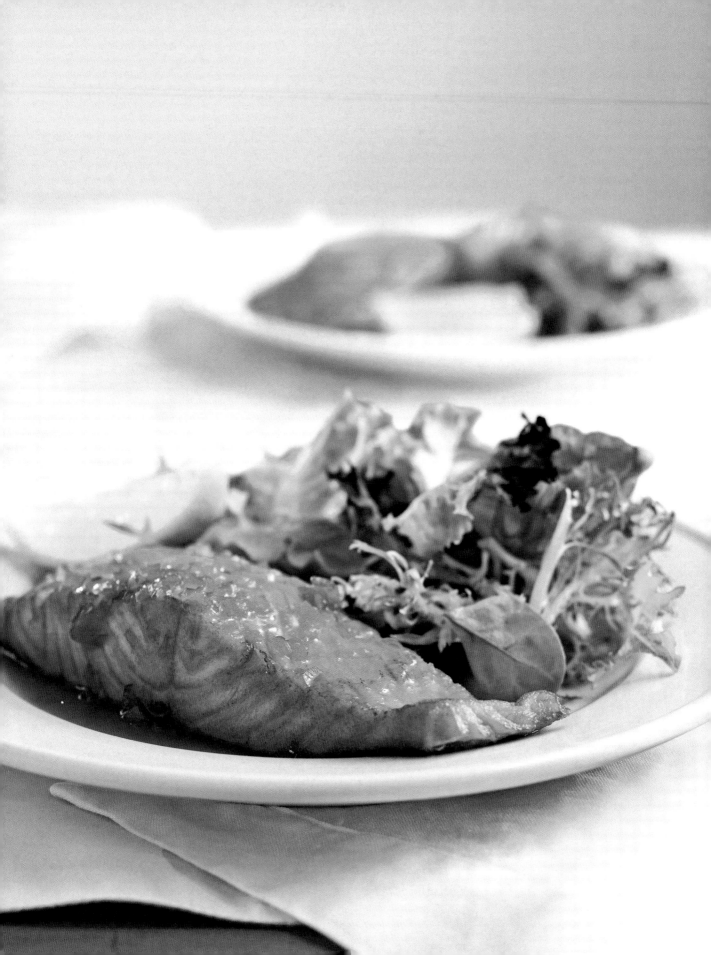

Pistachio-Crusted Tilapia Fillets

Meal total
286
CALORIES

125 ml (½ cup) plain breadcrumbs

80 ml (⅓ cup) unsalted pistachios, chopped

30 ml (2 tbsp) fresh dill, chopped

2.5 ml (½ tsp) fish seasoning

1 green onion, chopped

15 ml (1 tbsp) fresh parsley, chopped

4 tilapia fillets, 120 g (about ¼ lb) each

Prep time **15 minutes**

Cook time **12 minutes**

Serves **4**

PER SERVING	
Calories	204
Protein	27 g
Fat	7 g
Carbohydrates	9 g
Fibre	1 g
Iron	1 mg
Calcium	28 mg
Sodium	82 mg

1. Preheat the oven to 205°C (400°F).

2. In a bowl, mix the breadcrumbs with the pistachios, dill, fish seasoning, green onion and parsley.

3. Place the tilapia fillets on a baking sheet lined with parchment paper. Top the fish with the breadcrumb mix.

4. Bake for 12 to 15 minutes.

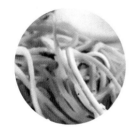

Try it with...

Saffron Julienne Vegetables
Per serving: 82 calories
Cut 2 zucchinis and 3 carrots into thin julienne strips. Heat 15 ml (1 tbsp) olive oil in a frying pan over medium heat. Cook 30 ml (2 tbsp) chopped shallots for 1 to 2 minutes. Pour 80 ml (⅓ cup) vegetable stock and add 4 to 5 saffron threads. Bring to a boil. Add the vegetables and cook for 4 to 5 minutes. Season with salt and pepper.

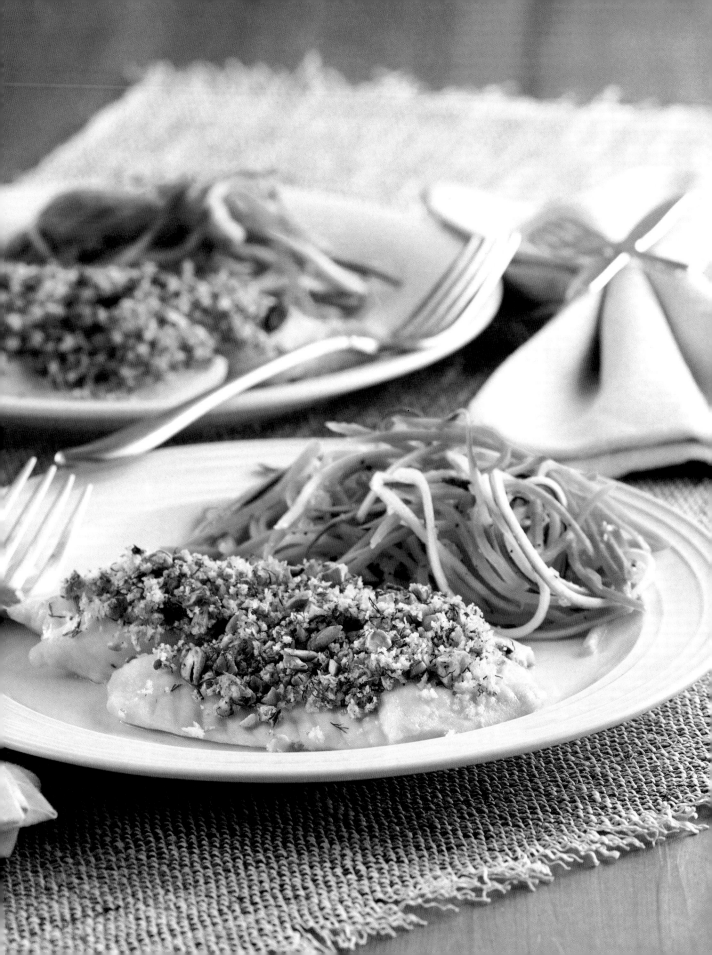

Fish Fillet With Baked Vegetables

Meal total
218
CALORIES

4 cod fillets, 150 g (⅓ lb) each

5 ml (1 tsp) salad seasoning

2 Italian tomatoes, sliced

½ yellow pepper, chopped

½ onion, chopped

1 garlic clove, minced

15 ml (1 tbsp) fresh parsley, chopped

15 ml (1 tbsp) fresh basil, chopped

125 ml (½ cup) pink grapefruit juice

180 ml (¾ cup) light cheddar, shredded

Prep time **20 minutes**

Cook time **20 minutes**

Serves **4**

PER SERVING	
Calories	218
Protein	34 g
Fat	5 g
Carbohydrates	8 g
Fibre	1 g
Iron	1 mg
Calcium	235 mg
Sodium	421 mg

1. Preheat the oven to 220°C (425°F).

2. Place the fish fillets side by side in an oiled baking dish. Sprinkle with salad seasoning.

3. Top the fillets with tomatoes, pepper, onion, garlic and herbs. Drizzle with grapefruit juice. Cover with cheese.

4. Bake for 20 to 25 minutes until the fish is fully cooked.

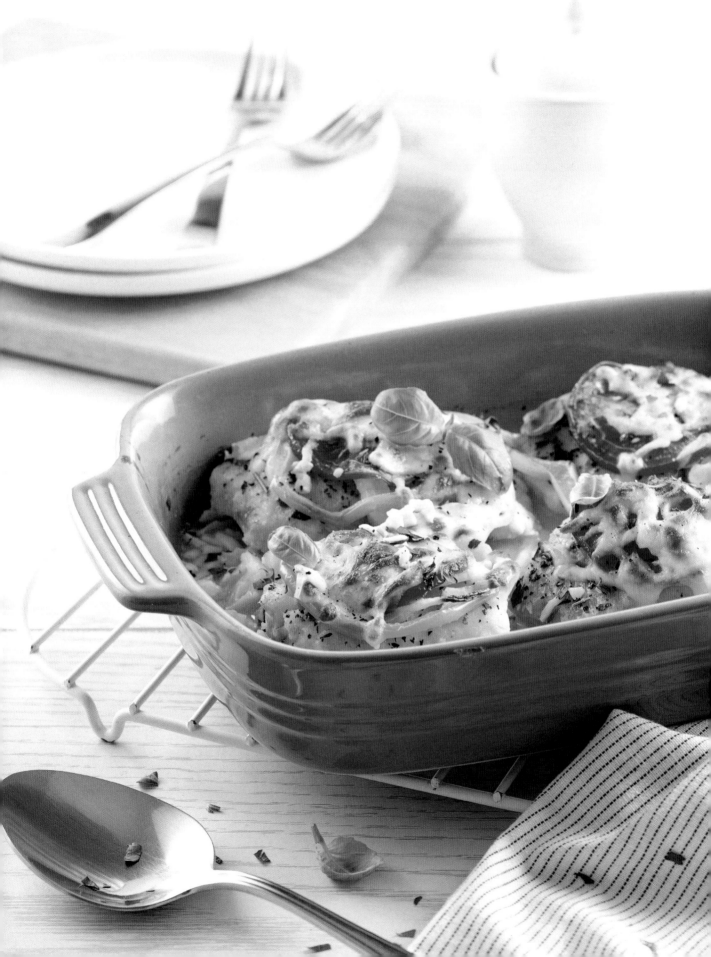

Salmon Teriyaki With Julienne Vegetables

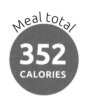

Meal total
352
CALORIES

4 salmon fillets, 100 g (3 ½ oz) each, skin removed

60 ml (¼ cup) teriyaki sauce

3 carrots, cut into thin julienne strips

2 zucchinis, cut into thin julienne strips

½ rutabaga, cut into thin julienne strips

15 ml (1 tbsp) sesame oil (untoasted)

1 onion, chopped

5 ml (1 tsp) garlic, minced

15 ml (1 tbsp) black and white sesame seeds

Prep time **15 minutes**

Cook time **18 minutes**

Serves **4**

PER SERVING	
Calories	352
Protein	25 g
Fat	19 g
Carbohydrates	20 g
Fibre	4 g
Iron	2 mg
Calcium	90 mg
Sodium	155 mg

1. Preheat the oven to 205°C (400°F).

2. Brush the salmon fillets with teriyaki sauce.

3. In a bowl, mix the julienne vegetables with the oil, onion and garlic.

4. Distribute the vegetable mix onto four large sheets of aluminum foil. Place a salmon fillet on each bed of vegetables. Sprinkle with sesame seeds. Fold up the foil, sealing the edges to form airtight packets. Place the packets on a baking sheet.

5. Bake for 18 to 20 minutes, until the packets are puffed and the fish flakes easily with a fork.

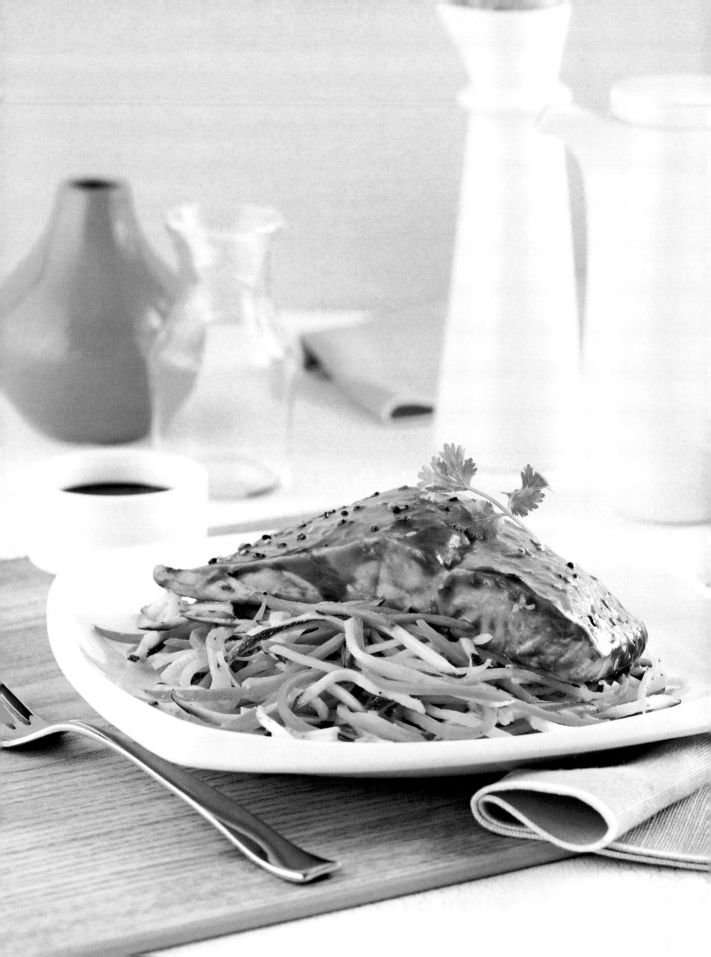

Salmon Edamame Stir-Fry

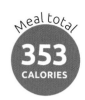

Meal total
353
CALORIES

500 ml (2 cups) frozen edamame (soybeans)

2 chopped green onions (optional)

For the stir-fry:

30 ml (2 tbsp) canola oil

400 g (about 1 lb) skinless salmon fillets, cut into cubes

For the sauce:

250 ml (1 cup) vegetable stock (no salt added)

60 ml (¼ cup) orange juice

30 ml (2 tbsp) honey

30 ml (2 tbsp) soy sauce (low-sodium)

15 ml (1 tbsp) ginger, minced

10 ml (2 tsp) garlic, minced

10 ml (2 tsp) orange zest

10 ml (2 tsp) cornstarch

2 star anise

Prep time **25 minutes**

Cook time **3 minutes**

Serves **4**

1. Cook the edamame according to the instructions on the packaging. Drain.

2. Mix the sauce ingredients in a bowl. Set aside.

3. Heat the oil in a frying pan or wok over medium-high heat. Sear the salmon cubes for 1 to 2 minutes on each surface, until they are golden-brown. Remove from the pan and set aside on a plate.

4. Pour the sauce into the same pan and add the edamame. Heat over medium heat until it starts to simmer, stirring. Add the salmon cubes and heat for 1 to 2 minutes.

5. Sprinkle each serving with green onions if desired.

PER SERVING	
Calories	353
Protein	31 g
Fat	18 g
Carbohydrates	24 g
Fibre	5 g
Iron	3 mg
Calcium	94 mg
Sodium	296 mg

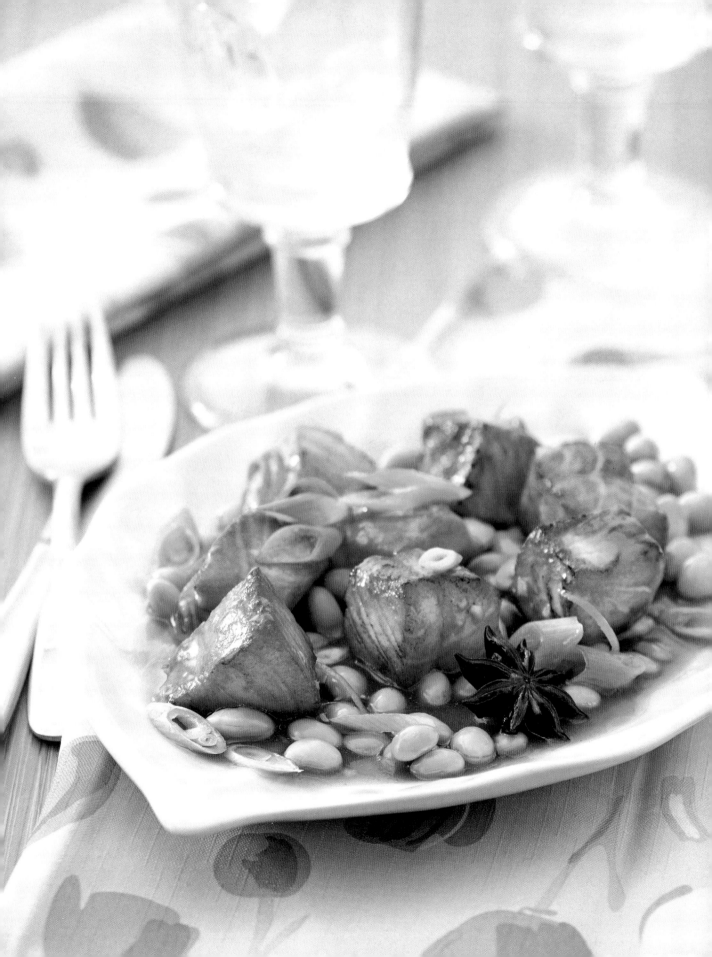

Pineapple-Glazed Shrimp

Meal total
282
CALORIES

1 can (398 ml) pineapple tidbits

15 ml (1 tbsp) honey

15 ml (1 tbsp) lime zest

24 medium shrimp (31-40 count), raw and peeled

7.5 ml (½ tbsp) canola oil

3 pepper halves, various colours, cut into cubes

½ red onion, chopped

16 sugar snap peas

Prep time **15 minutes**

Cook time **9 minutes**

Serves **4**

PER SERVING	
Calories	208
Protein	17 g
Fat	3 g
Carbohydrates	28 g
Fibre	2 g
Iron	3 mg
Calcium	73 mg
Sodium	120 mg

1. Pour the pineapple juice from the can into a bowl. Mix with the honey, lime zest and shrimp. Let marinate in the refrigerator for 8 to 10 minutes.

2. Drain the shrimp, setting aside the marinade.

3. Heat the oil in a frying pan over medium heat. Cook the shrimp for 2 minutes on each side. Set aside on a plate.

4. In the same pan, cook the pineapple, peppers, red onion and snap peas for 3 to 4 minutes.

5. Add the shrimp and the reserved marinade to the pan. Cook for 2 to 3 minutes, until the shrimp caramelize.

Try it with...

Almond Milk-Flavoured Rice
Per serving: 74 calories
Rinse 125 ml (½ cup) jasmine rice in cold water. Place in a pot with 200 ml (about ¾ cup) almond milk, 125 ml (½ cup) water and a pinch of salt. Bring to a boil. Cover and cook over medium-low heat for 20 to 25 minutes, stirring from time to time, until the rice is cooked.

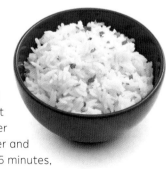

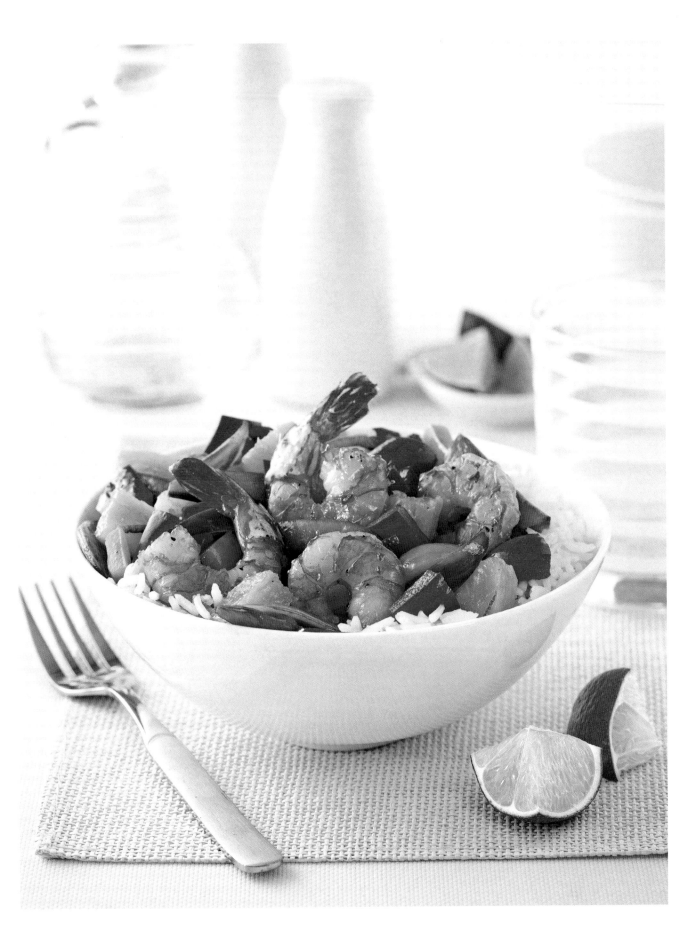

Five-Spice Shrimp Stir-Fry

Meal total

362 CALORIES

125 ml (½ cup) white rice

2.5 ml (½ tsp) Chinese five-spice blend

200 ml (about ¾ cup) orange and ginger stir-fry sauce

15 ml (1 tbsp) canola oil

350 g (about ¾ lb) shrimp (31-40 count), raw and peeled

½ bag (750 g) frozen mixed stir-fry vegetables

30 ml (2 tbsp) honey

½ can (540 ml) mandarin oranges, drained

2 green onions, chopped

Prep time **15 minutes**

Cook time **15 minutes**

Serves **4**

PER SERVING	
Calories	362
Protein	17 g
Fat	5 g
Carbohydrates	64 g
Fibre	5 g
Iron	4 mg
Calcium	81 mg
Sodium	917 mg

1. Cook the rice according to the instructions on the packaging.

2. In a bowl, mix the Chinese five-spice blend with the orange and ginger sauce.

3. Heat the oil in a wok or frying pan over medium heat. Cook the shrimp for 1 minute on each side. Transfer the shrimp onto a plate.

4. In the same wok, cook the vegetables for 2 to 3 minutes, until tender.

5. Pour in the sauce and the honey. Bring to a boil. Put the shrimp back into the wok. Add the mandarin oranges and stir.

6. Distribute the rice onto plates and top with the shrimp preparation. Sprinkle each serving with green onions.

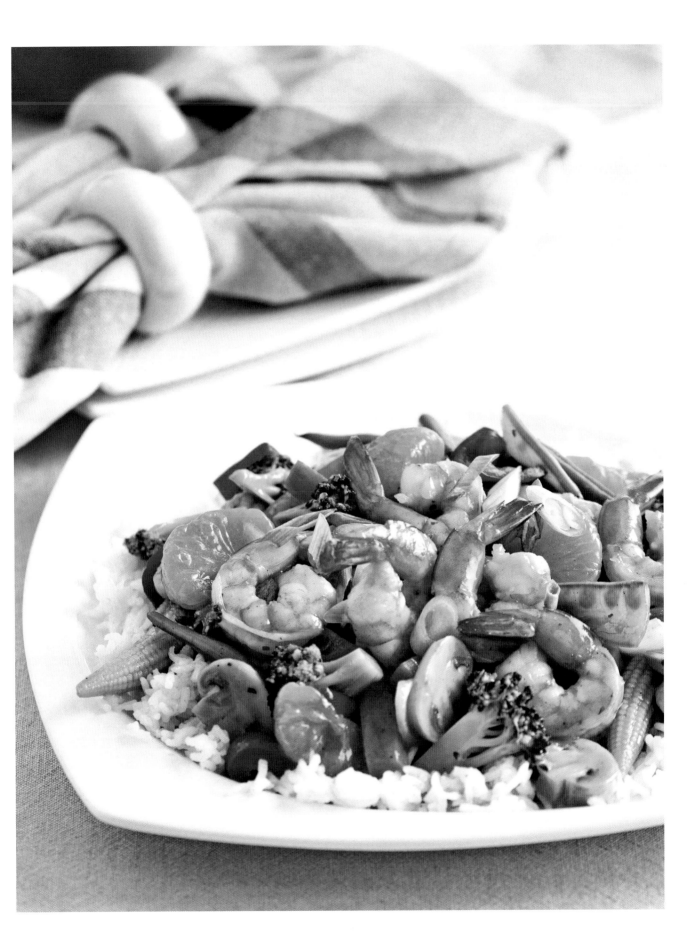

Sole Rolls With Asparagus

Meal total

299
CALORIES

24 asparagus spears

8 sole fillets, 80 g (about ⅕ lb) each

Salt and pepper to taste

60 ml (¼ cup) grated Parmesan

125 ml (½ cup) mascarpone

80 ml (⅓ cup) milk

45 ml (3 tbsp) sun-dried tomato pesto

15 ml (1 tbsp) lemon zest

Prep time **15 minutes**

Cook time **17 minutes**

Serves **4**

PER SERVING	
Calories	299
Protein	27 g
Fat	18 g
Carbohydrates	7 g
Fibre	3 g
Iron	3 mg
Calcium	178 mg
Sodium	681 mg

1. Preheat the oven to 190°C (375°F).

2. Blanch the asparagus for 2 to 3 minutes in boiling, salted water. Submerge in ice water and then drain.

3. Place three asparagus spears onto each sole fillet. Season with salt and pepper. Roll up the sole fillets around the asparagus. Place the rolls on a baking sheet lined with parchment paper. Sprinkle with Parmesan. Bake for 15 to 20 minutes.

4. While the sole is cooking, prepare the sauce by heating the mascarpone with the milk, pesto and lemon zest in a pot. Season with salt and pepper. Let simmer over low heat for 2 to 3 minutes. Serve with the fish.

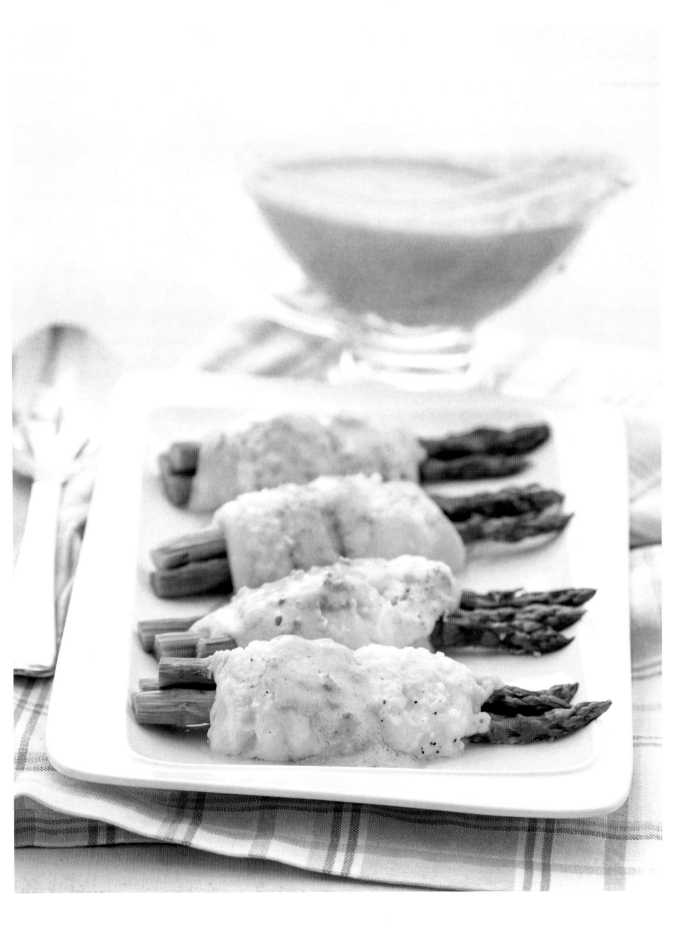

Gourmet Meat

Veal stir-fry, maple molasses pork tenderloin, steak with shallots... who said anything about healthy eating being boring? Here are 13 gourmet dishes that meat lovers can savour without the guilt... or the fat!

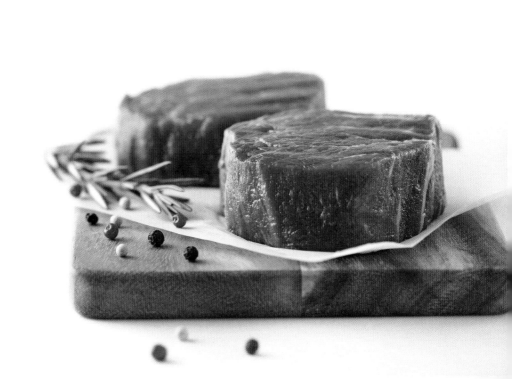

Orange Beef Stir-Fry

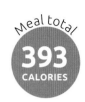

160 ml (⅔ cup) white rice

125 ml (½ cup) teriyaki marinade (low-sodium)

15 ml (1 tbsp) cornstarch

125 ml (½ cup) orange juice

10 ml (2 tsp) orange zest

15 ml (1 tbsp) canola oil

450 g (1 lb) beef sirloin, cut into strips

½ red pepper, cut into cubes

½ yellow pepper, cut into cubes

1 onion, chopped

30 ml (2 tbsp) honey

1 green onion, chopped

Prep time **15 minutes**

Cook time **15 minutes**

Serves **4**

PER SERVING	
Calories	393
Protein	30 g
Fat	8 g
Carbohydrates	50 g
Fibre	2 g
Iron	4 mg
Calcium	29 mg
Sodium	747 mg

1. Cook the rice according to the instructions on the packaging.

2. While the rice is cooking, mix the teriyaki marinade with the cornstarch and the orange juice and zest.

3. Heat the oil in a frying pan over medium heat. Sear the beef strips for 1 to 2 minutes on each side.

4. Add the peppers and onion. Cook for 1 to 2 minutes.

5. Add the honey and the prepared sauce. Bring to a boil and cook for another 2 minutes.

6. Serve with the rice and sprinkle each serving with green onions.

Also try it...

With Homemade Teriyaki Sauce

It's easy to make teriyaki sauce at home. Add 250 ml (1 cup) low-sodium soy sauce, 125 ml (½ cup) brown sugar, 45 ml (3 tbsp) mirin and 30 ml (2 tbsp) chicken stock to a pot and bring to a boil. Reduce to low heat as soon as it starts to simmer. Let simmer for 5 minutes.

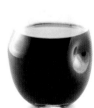

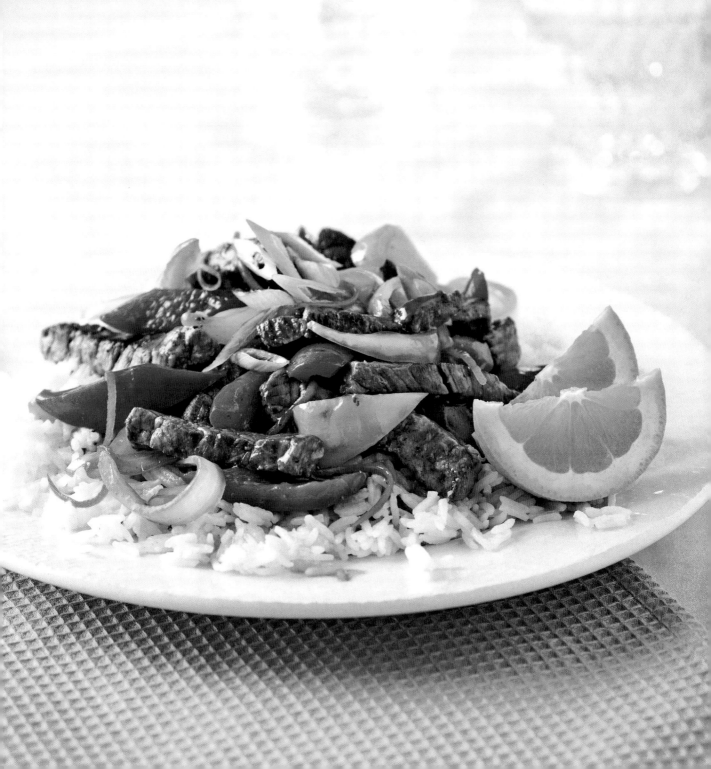

Veal Cutlets With Pepper Marsala Sauce

Meal total
398
CALORIES

15 ml (1 tbsp) canola oil

4 veal cutlets, 120 g
(about ¼ lb) each

60 ml (¼ cup) shallots, chopped

10 mushrooms, sliced

80 ml (⅓ cup) Marsala wine

310 ml (1 ¼ cups)
pepper sauce

30 ml (2 tbsp) fresh chives,
chopped

Prep time **20 minutes**

Cook time **5 minutes**

Serves **4**

PER SERVING	
Calories	265
Protein	31 g
Fat	7 g
Carbohydrates	15 g
Fibre	1 g
Iron	2 mg
Calcium	16 mg
Sodium	682 mg

1. Heat the oil in a frying pan over medium heat. Cook the veal cutlets for 1 minute on each side. Transfer to a plate and cover with aluminum foil.

2. In the same pan, cook the shallots and mushrooms for 1 to 2 minutes.

3. Add the Marsala wine and pepper sauce. Bring to a boil. Put the cutlets back into the pan and heat for 2 to 3 minutes over low heat.

4. Serve the cutlets onto plates and top with the sauce. Sprinkle each serving with chives.

Try it with...

Creamy Herb and Parmesan Polenta
Per serving: 133 calories
Pour 480 ml (about 2 cups) milk into a pot and bring to a boil over medium heat. Sprinkle 80 ml (⅓ cup) cornmeal into the pot, whisking until it thickens. Cook over low heat for 15 minutes. Add 45 ml (3 tbsp) grated Parmesan, 15 ml (1 tbsp) fresh chives, chopped, and 15 ml (1 tbsp) fresh parsley, chopped. Season with salt and pepper.

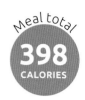

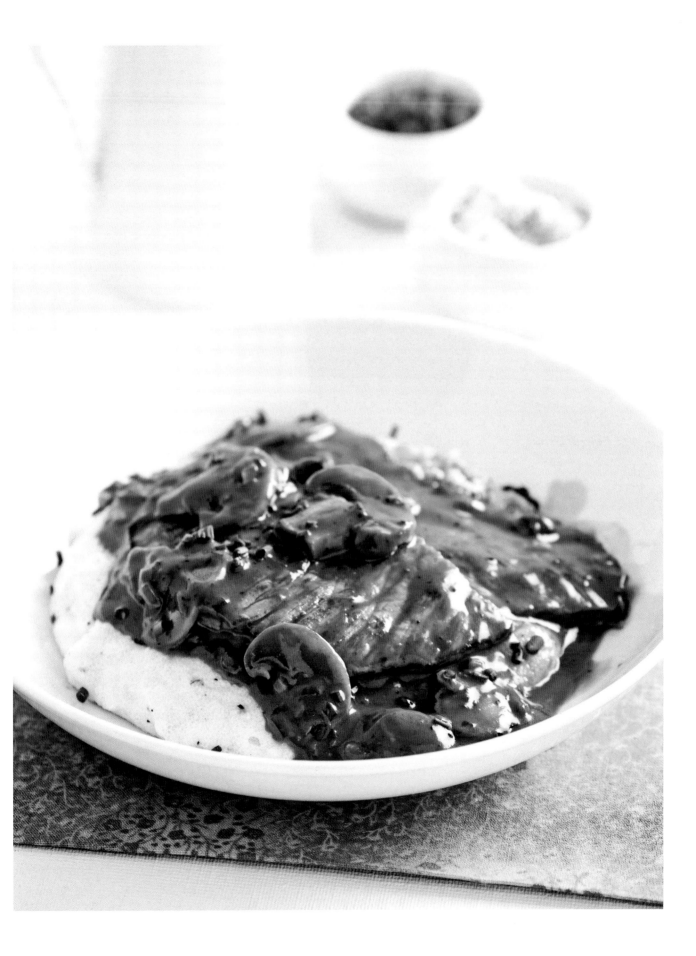

Veal Navarin

8 carrots, with the tops

12 creamer potatoes, peeled

12 red pearl onions

15 ml (1 tbsp) olive oil

675 g (about 1 ½ lb) veal cubes

15 ml (1 tbsp) garlic, minced

45 ml (3 tbsp) flour

60 ml (¼ cup) tomato paste

1 litre (4 cups) beef stock (low-sodium)

1 sprig thyme

1 bay leaf

1 sprig rosemary

Pepper to taste

100 g (3 ½ oz) green beans

250 ml (1 cup) green peas

45 ml (3 tbsp) flat-leaf parsley

Prep time **30 minutes**

Cook time **2 hours 20 minutes**

Serves **6**

PER SERVING	
Calories	356
Protein	33 g
Fat	6 g
Carbohydrates	44 g
Fibre	10 g
Iron	4 mg
Calcium	112 mg
Sodium	206 mg

1. Peel the carrots, creamer potatoes and pearl onions.

2. Heat the oil in a pot over medium heat. Sear a few veal cubes at a time for 3 to 4 minutes on each side, until they are golden-brown. Set aside on a plate.

3. Cook the garlic in a pot for 30 minutes. Add the veal cubes and flour. Stir. Stir in the tomato paste. Add the stock and herbs. Season with pepper. Bring to a boil, and then cover and cook for 1 hour over low heat.

4. Add the carrots, potatoes and onions. Cook for another 37 to 45 minutes, until the meat is no longer pink in the centre.

5. Add the green beans and peas to the pot and cook for another 5 to 8 minutes.

6. Sprinkle each serving with parsley leaves.

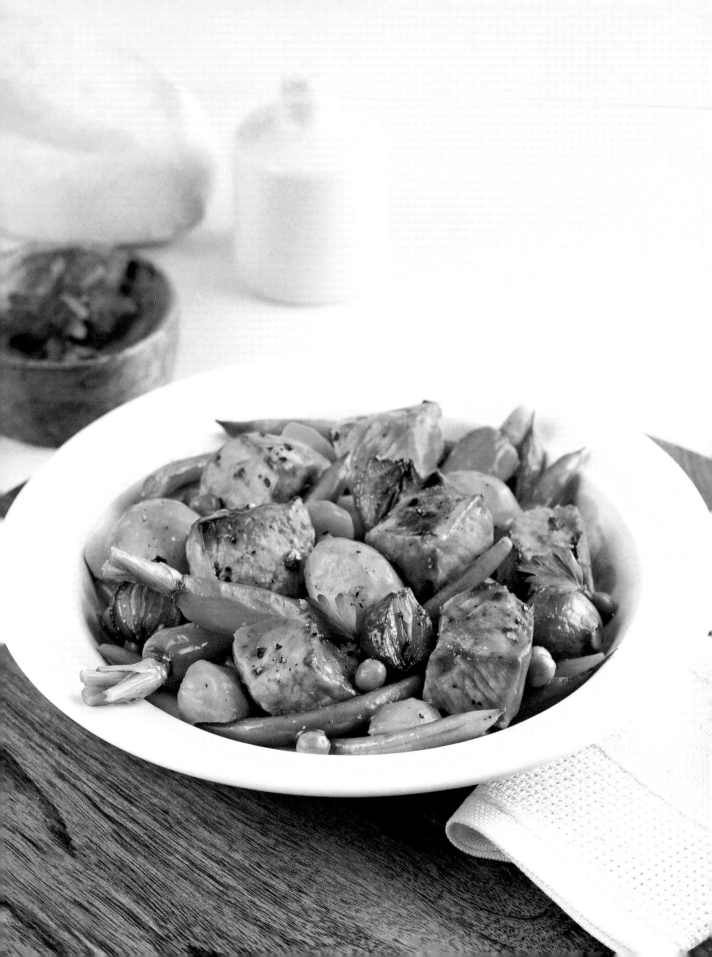

Maple Molasses Pork Tenderloin

Meal total
397
CALORIES

680 g (1 ½ lb) pork tenderloins

15 ml (1 tbsp) canola oil

45 ml (3 tbsp) shallots, chopped

15 ml (1 tbsp) flour

For the maple molasses sauce:

250 ml (1 cup) chicken stock

80 ml (⅓ cup) maple syrup

30 ml (2 tbsp) molasses

15 ml (1 tbsp) Dijon mustard

Salt and pepper to taste

Prep time **15 minutes**

Cook time **20 minutes**

Serves **4**

PER SERVING	
Calories	325
Protein	39 g
Fat	6 g
Carbohydrates	27 g
Fibre	0 g
Iron	4 mg
Calcium	139 mg
Sodium	368 mg

1. Trim the pork tenderloins by removing the silver skin.

2. Whisk together the sauce ingredients in a bowl. Set aside.

3. Heat the oil in a frying pan over medium heat. Sear the pork tenderloins on all sides until they are golden-brown. Transfer to a plate.

4. In the same pan, cook the shallots for 1 minute. Sprinkle with the flour and stir. Add the maple molasses sauce. Cover and cook for 20 minutes over medium-low heat.

5. Transfer the pork tenderloins to a plate. Cover with aluminum foil and let rest for 5 to 8 minutes before slicing them. Serve with the sauce.

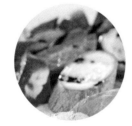

Try it with...

Sautéed Vegetables
Per serving: 72 calories
Slice 2 zucchinis, cut 2 carrots lengthwise and dice 1 red pepper. Heat 15 ml (1 tbsp) olive oil in a frying pan over medium heat. Sauté the vegetables until they are tender, stirring from time to time. Season with salt and pepper.

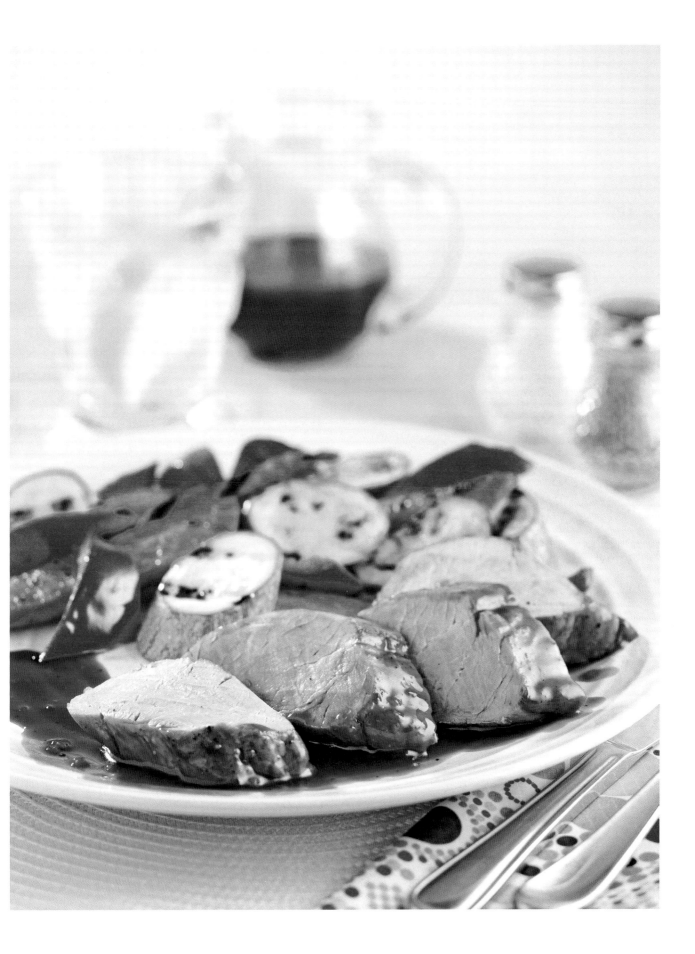

Pork Stew With Mustard Sauce

Meal total
394
CALORIES

15 ml (1 tbsp) canola oil

680 g (1 ½ lb) pork cubes for stew

125 ml (½ cup) 15 % cooking cream

For the sauce:

750 ml (3 cups) vegetable stock

60 ml (¼ cup) flour

45 ml (3 tbsp) Dijon mustard

30 ml (2 tbsp) whole-grain mustard

15 ml (1 tbsp) fresh thyme, chopped

2 onions, chopped

Salt and pepper to taste

Prep time **15 minutes**

Cook time **50 minutes**

Serves **6**

PER SERVING	
Calories	328
Protein	25 g
Fat	21 g
Carbohydrates	8 g
Fibre	1 g
Iron	2 mg
Calcium	54 mg
Sodium	399 mg

1. Preheat the oven to 190°C (375°F).

2. Mix the sauce ingredients in a large bowl.

3. Heat the oil in a Dutch oven or ovenproof saucepan over medium heat. Brown the pork cubes for a few minutes. Transfer the meat to a plate and throw out the cooking oil.

4. Put the meat back into the Dutch oven and add the sauce. Cover and bake for 45 minutes.

5. Remove from the oven and add the cream. Let simmer on the stove for 5 minutes over low heat.

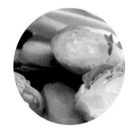

Try it with...

Brussel Sprouts and Carrots
Per serving: 66 calories
Place a steamer basket in a pot. Add water to the bottom of the pot. Cut 20 Brussel sprouts in half and cut 4 carrots into diagonal slices. Place in the steamer basket with 2 sprigs of thyme. Bring the water to a boil and let the vegetables steam for 10 to 12 minutes. Season with salt and pepper before serving.

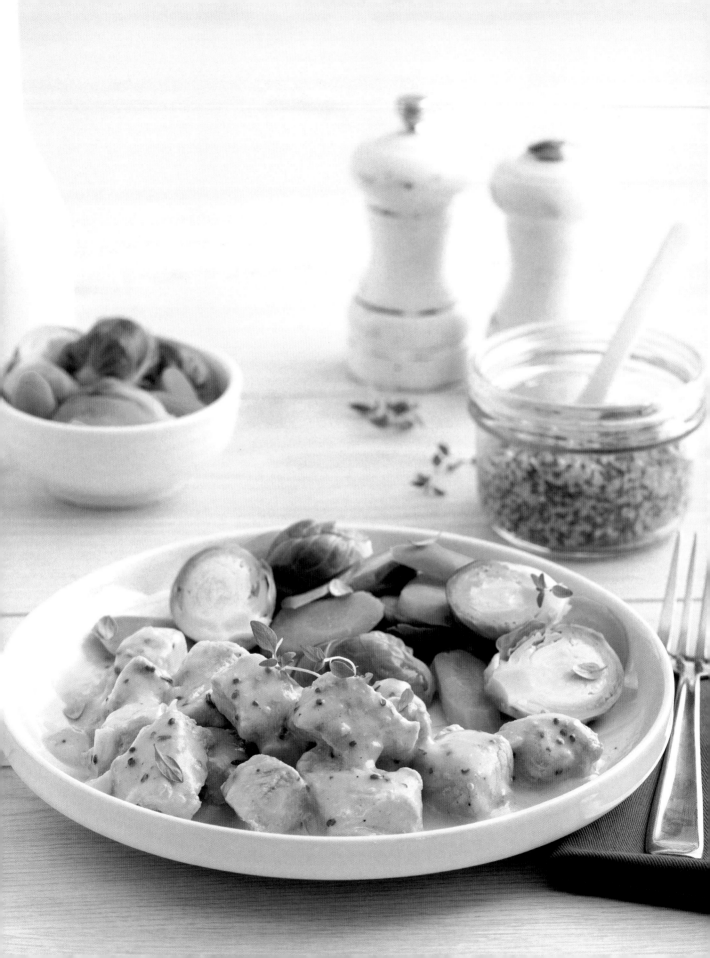

Cabbage Rolls Casserole

Meal total
347
CALORIES

12 large Savoy cabbage leaves

15 ml (1 tbsp) olive oil

675 g (1 ½ lb) lean ground veal

1 onion, chopped

15 ml (1 tbsp) garlic, minced

1 can (540 ml) diced tomatoes

250 ml (1 cup) parboiled long grain brown rice

250 ml (1 cup) beef stock (low-sodium)

60 ml (¼ cup) chopped parsley

Salt and pepper to taste

750 ml (3 cups) tomato sauce (no salt added)

Prep time **25 minutes**

Cook time **51 minutes**

Serves **8**

PER SERVING	
Calories	347
Protein	22 g
Fat	14 g
Carbohydrates	34 g
Fibre	5 g
Iron	7 mg
Calcium	59 mg
Sodium	351 mg

1. Preheat the oven to 205°C (400°F).

2. Cook the cabbage leaves in a pot of boiling, salted water for 5 minutes. Rinse under cold water and drain.

3. In the same pot, heat the oil in a pot over medium heat. Cook the ground veal for 5 to 7 minutes, breaking up the meat with a wooden spoon, until it is no longer pink.

4. Add the onion and garlic. Cook for another 1 minute.

5. Add the diced tomatoes, rice and stock. Bring to a boil.

6. Take off the stove and add the parsley. Season with salt and pepper, and stir.

7. Spread a little bit of the tomato sauce over the bottom of a 33 cm x 23 cm (13 in x 9 in) baking dish. Cover with 4 cabbage leaves, half of the meat preparation and half of the remaining tomato sauce. Repeat once, and cover with the last 4 cabbage leaves.

8. Cover the dish with a sheet of aluminum foil. Bake for 40 to 50 minutes, until the rice is cooked.

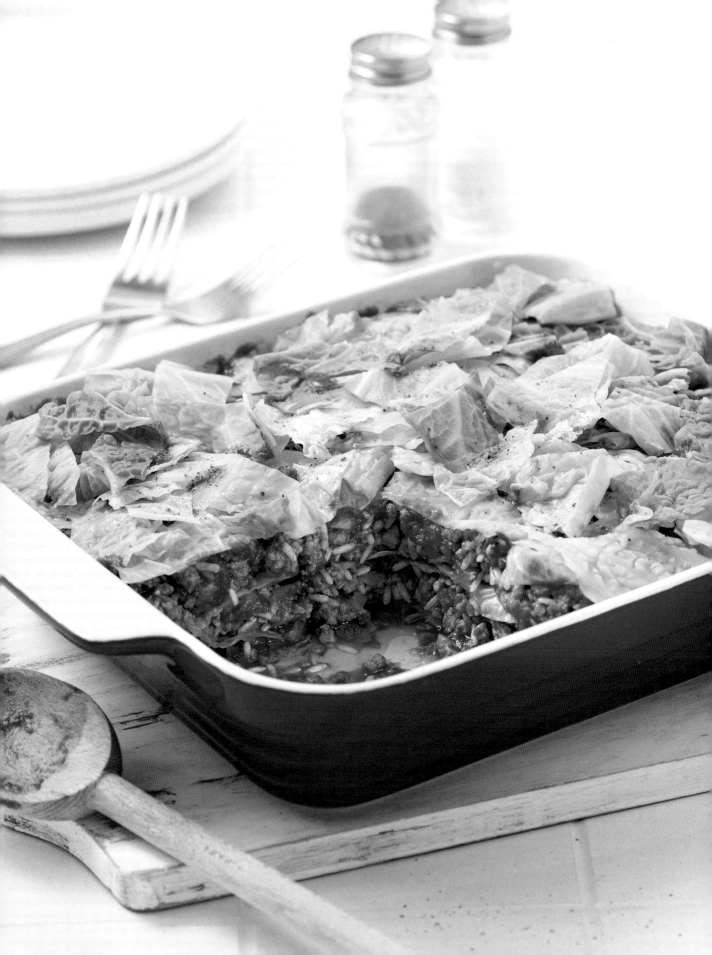

Steak With Red Wine Sauce

Meal total
383
CALORIES

4 strip loin steaks,
150 g (⅓ lb) each

15 ml (1 tbsp) olive oil

15 ml (1 tbsp) butter

4 shallots, chopped

60 ml (¼ cup) red wine

1 can (284 ml) beef consommé

10 ml (2 tsp) pink peppercorns

Salt to taste

10 ml (2 tsp) cornstarch

Prep time **20 minutes**

Cook time **6 minutes**

Serves **4**

PER SERVING	
Calories	315
Protein	39 g
Fat	13 g
Carbohydrates	5 g
Fibre	1 g
Iron	4 mg
Calcium	24 mg
Sodium	567 mg

1. Let the beef steaks rest at room temperature for 15 to 20 minutes before cooking.

2. Heat the oil and butter in a frying pan over medium-high heat. Sear the steaks for 1 to 2 minutes on each side. Set aside on a plate.

3. In the same pan, cook the shallots for 3 to 4 minutes, until they are golden-brown and tender.

4. Add the wine, consommé, pink peppercorns and salt. Let simmer over medium heat for 1 to 2 minutes.

5. Dissolve the cornstarch in a little cold water and pour it into the pan. Stir until it thickens.

6. Add the steaks and heat for 1 minute.

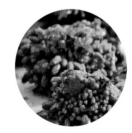

Try it with...

Sautéed Sun-Dried Tomato Pesto Rapini
Per serving: 68 calories
Blanch 1 bunch rapini in boiling, salted water for 2 to 3 minutes. Drain and cut into pieces. Heat 15 ml (1 tbsp) butter and 15 ml (1 tbsp) sun-dried tomato pesto in a frying pan over medium heat. Add the rapini and cook for 3 to 4 minutes, stirring from time to time. Season with salt and pepper.

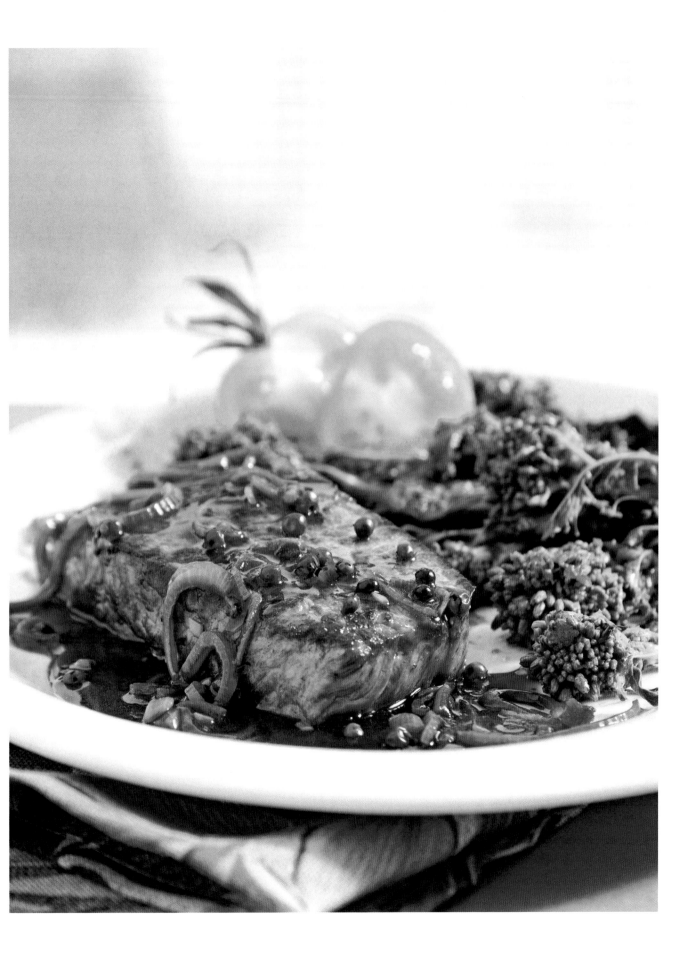

Quinoa and Beef Stuffed Peppers

Meal total
388
CALORIES

4 small peppers,
various colours

15 ml (1 tbsp) olive oil

300 g (⅔ lb) extra-lean
ground beef

1 onion, chopped

15 ml (1 tbsp) garlic, minced

1 zucchini, diced

15 ml (1 tbsp) Italian seasoning

160 ml (⅔ cup)
marinara sauce

430 ml (1 ¾ cups)
cooked quinoa

Salt and pepper to taste

4 small Italian tomatoes, diced

125 ml (½ cup) light mozzarella,
shredded

30 ml (2 tbsp) small basil leaves

Prep time **15 minutes**

Cook time **33 minutes**

Serves **4**

PER SERVING	
Calories	388
Protein	26 g
Fat	16 g
Carbohydrates	35 g
Fibre	7 g
Iron	4 mg
Calcium	194 mg
Sodium	336 mg

1. Preheat the oven to 180°C (350°F).

2. Slice off the top third of the peppers and remove the white membranes and seeds. Place on a baking sheet lined with parchment paper.

3. Heat the olive oil in a large frying pan over medium heat. Cook the ground beef for 5 to 7 minutes, breaking up the meat with a wooden spoon.

4. Add the onion, garlic, zucchini and Italian seasoning. Cook for another 3 to 4 minutes.

5. Add the marinara sauce and cooked quinoa. Season with salt and pepper, and stir.

6. Stuff the peppers with the prepared beef. Top with tomatoes and cheese.

7. Bake for 25 to 30 minutes.

8. Sprinkle each serving with basil.

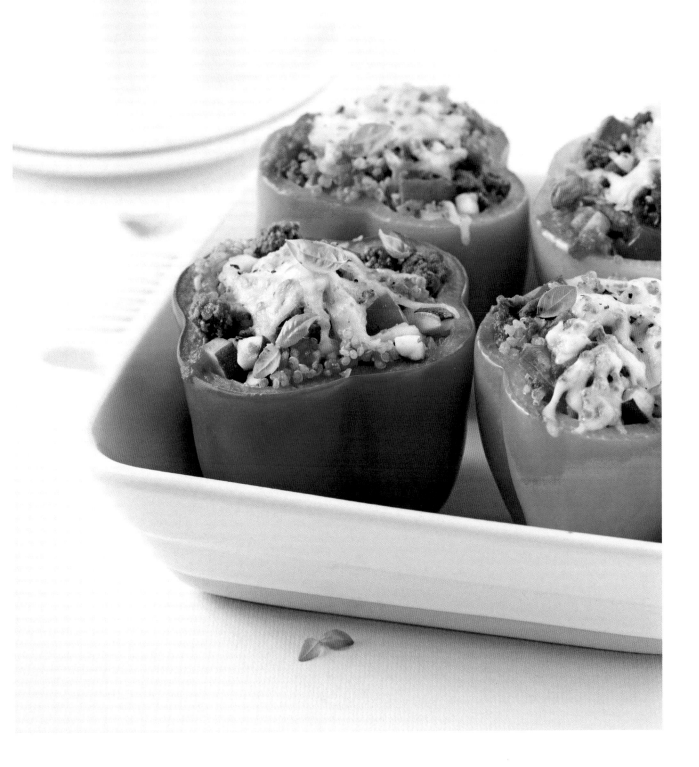

Mini Meatloaves With Salsa

Meal total
270
CALORIES

1 egg

125 ml (½ cup) oats

450 g (1 lb) extra-lean ground beef

30 ml (2 tbsp) chili sauce

125 ml (½ cup) salsa

Salt and pepper to taste

30 ml (2 tbsp) ketchup

Prep time **15 minutes**

Cook time **27 minutes**

Serves **4**

PER SERVING	
Calories	270
Protein	27 g
Fat	11 g
Carbohydrates	14 g
Fibre	2 g
Iron	3 mg
Calcium	28 mg
Sodium	467 mg

1. Preheat the oven to 205°C (400°F).

2. In a bowl, mix the egg with the oats, ground beef, chili sauce and half of the salsa. Season with salt and pepper.

3. Form four patties with the prepared meat and place on a baking sheet lined with parchment paper. Bake for 15 minutes.

4. While the patties are cooking, mix the rest of the salsa with the ketchup.

5. Remove the baking sheet from the oven. Spread the ketchup mixture over the patties. Bake for another 12 to 15 minutes, until the mini meatloaves are no longer pink in the centre.

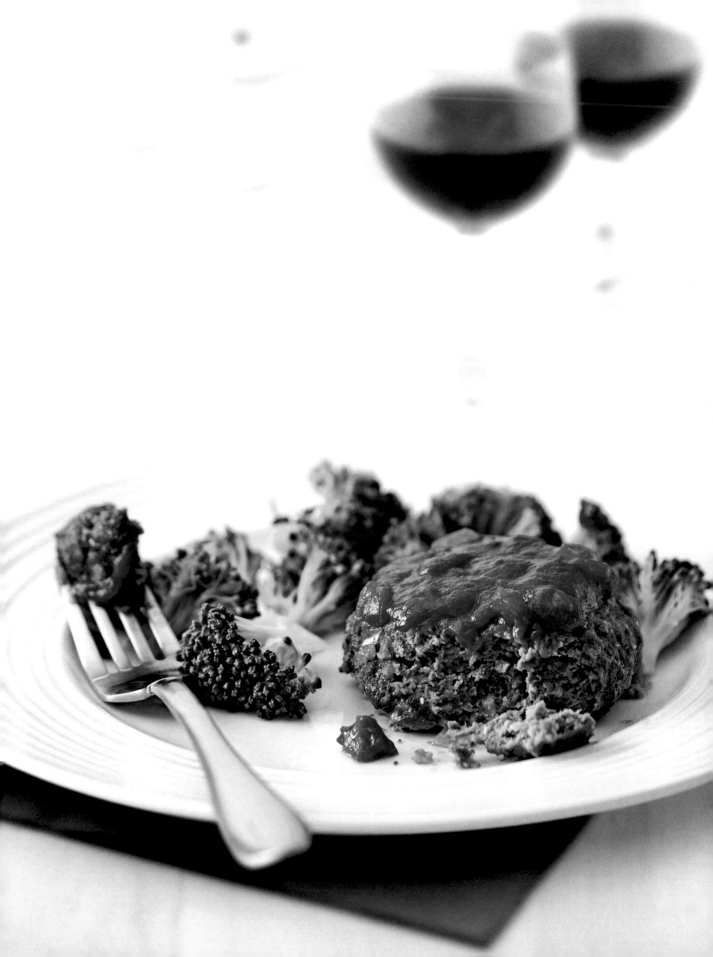

Chili

20 ml (4 tsp) olive oil

1 kg (about 2 ¼ lb) extra-lean ground beef

1 ½ onions, chopped

45 ml (3 tbsp) chili powder

15 ml (1 tbsp) garlic, minced

375 ml (1 ½ cups) corn kernels

1 ½ cans (796 ml each) diced tomatoes

20 to 25 cherry tomatoes, cut in half

4 peppers, various colours, diced

Salt and pepper to taste

125 ml (½ cup) cilantro leaves

Prep time **20 minutes**

Cook time **18 minutes**

Serves **8**

PER SERVING	
Calories	339
Protein	31 g
Fat	13 g
Carbohydrates	28 g
Fibre	4 g
Iron	5 mg
Calcium	96 mg
Sodium	513 mg

1. Heat the oil in a large frying pan over medium heat. Cook the ground beef and onions for 8 to 10 minutes, breaking up the meat with a wooden spoon, until it is no longer pink.

2. Stir in the chili powder, garlic, corn and diced tomatoes. Cook for another 10 to 12 minutes.

3. Add the cherry tomatoes and peppers. Season with salt and pepper. Stir gently.

4. Serve the chili into bowls. Sprinkle with cilantro.

Try it with...

Toasted Pita Chips
Per serving: 61 calories
Cut 3 medium pitas into eight wedges and place on a baking sheet. Bake for 8 to 10 minutes at 190°C (375°F) until crispy, turning them over at the halfway point.

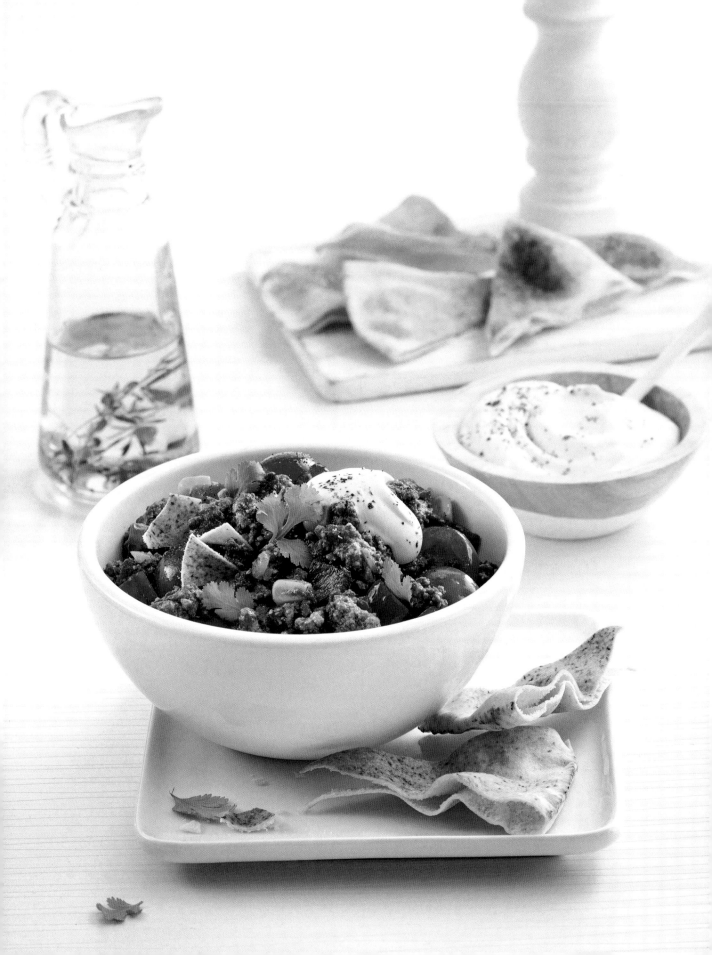

Veal and Mushroom Stew

15 ml (1 tbsp) canola oil

755 g (1 ⅔ lb) veal cubes

2 onions, chopped

3 carrots, diced

45 ml (3 tbsp) unbleached
all-purpose flour

30 ml (2 tbsp) Dijon mustard

750 ml (3 cups) chicken stock
(no salt added)

250 ml (1 cup) white wine

Salt and pepper to taste

10 white mushrooms

10 shiitakes

6 oyster mushrooms

30 ml (2 tbsp) fresh tarragon,
chopped

Prep time **25 minutes**

Cook time **45 minutes**

Serves **6**

PER SERVING	
Calories	324
Protein	35 g
Fat	8 g
Carbohydrates	25 g
Fibre	6 g
Iron	4 mg
Calcium	60 mg
Sodium	301 mg

1. Heat the oil in a pot or Dutch oven over medium-high heat. Brown the veal cubes with the onions for 2 to 3 minutes.

2. Add the carrots. Sprinkle with flour and stir. Add the mustard, stock and wine. Season with salt and pepper. Cover and let simmer for 30 minutes over low heat.

3. While the veal is cooking, slice the mushrooms.

4. Add the mushrooms and tarragon to the pot. Cook about 15 more minutes, until the meat is tender.

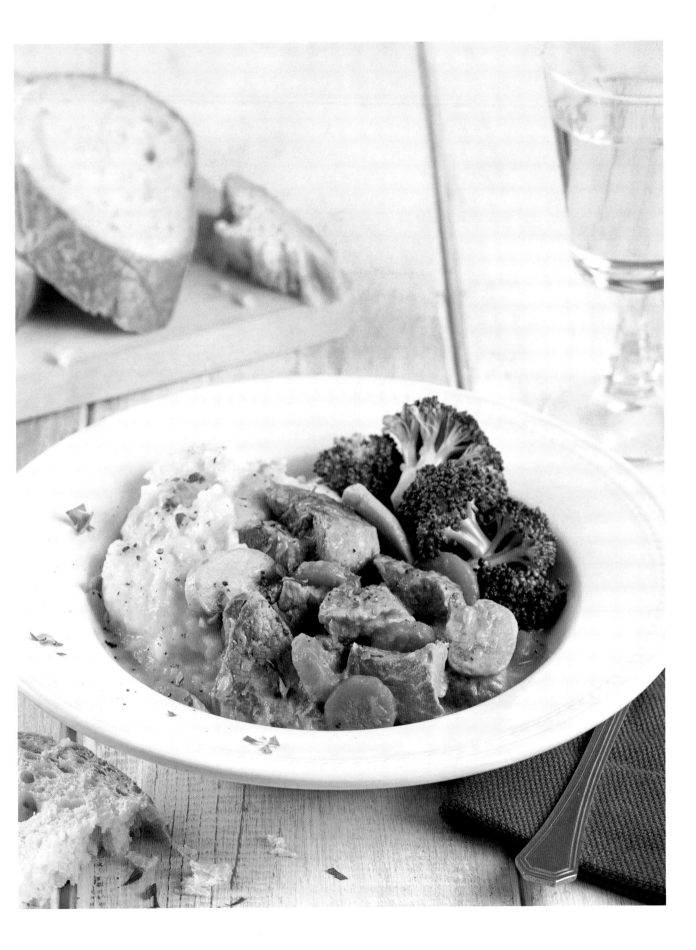

Asian Veal Stir-Fry

60 ml (¼ cup) cornstarch

600 g (about 1 ⅓ lb) veal cutlets, cut into strips

15 ml (1 tbsp) canola oil

1 onion, chopped

5 ml (1 tsp) garlic, minced

1 carrot, chopped

250 ml (1 cup) snow peas

250 ml (1 cup) beef stock (no salt added)

30 ml (2 tbsp) soy sauce (low-sodium)

30 ml (2 tbsp) honey

125 ml (½ cup) bean sprouts

Prep time **15 minutes**

Cook time **7 minutes**

Serves **4**

PER SERVING	
Calories	307
Protein	37 g
Fat	6 g
Carbohydrates	26 g
Fibre	2 g
Iron	3 mg
Calcium	49 mg
Sodium	585 mg

1. Put the cornstarch into an airtight bag. Add the veal strips to the bag and shake it to fully coat the meat.

2. Heat the oil in a frying pan or wok over medium-high heat. Brown a few veal strips at a time for 2 minutes. Remove from the pan and set aside on a plate.

3. In the same pan, sear the onion and garlic for 1 minute.

4. Add the carrot, snow peas, stock, soy sauce and honey. Heat until it starts to simmer and cook for 1 minute.

5. Put the veal back into the pan and add the bean sprouts. Cook for 2 to 3 minutes.

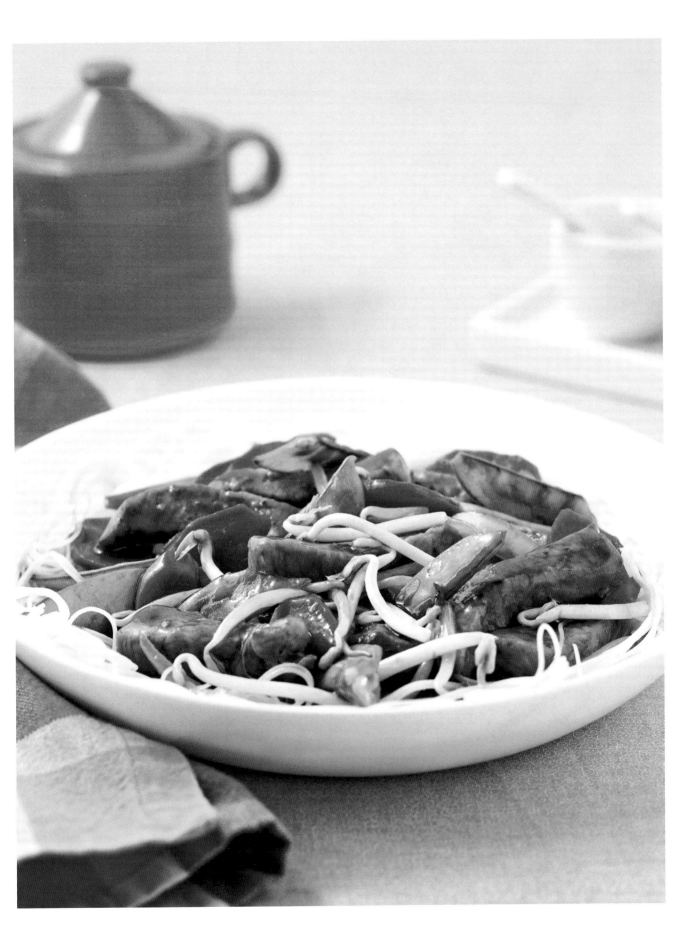

Meatball and Vegetable Stew

Meal total
318
CALORIES

450 g (1 lb) lean ground beef

1 onion, chopped

1 egg

30 ml (2 tbsp) fresh parsley, chopped

15 ml (1 tbsp) fresh thyme, chopped

15 ml (1 tbsp) butter

1 ½ cans (284 ml each) beef consommé

500 ml (2 cups) frozen diced vegetable mix

4 potatoes, peeled and diced

125 ml (½ cup) red wine

Prep time **15 minutes**

Cook time **18 minutes**

Serves **4**

PER SERVING	
Calories	262
Protein	22 g
Fat	9 g
Carbohydrates	23 g
Fibre	6 g
Iron	3 mg
Calcium	64 mg
Sodium	224 mg

1. In a bowl, mix the ground beef with the onion, egg and herbs.

2. Form balls using about 30 ml (2 tbsp) of the prepared beef for each one.

3. Melt the butter in a pot over medium heat. Brown the meatballs on all sides.

4. Add the beef consommé, vegetables, potatoes and red wine. Cover and cook for 18 to 20 minutes over medium-high heat, until the meatballs are no longer pink in the centre.

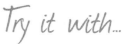

Try it with...

Mâche, Curly Leaf Lettuce and Artichoke Salad
Per serving: 56 calories
In a salad bowl, mix 15 ml (1 tbsp) olive oil with 30 ml (2 tbsp) lemon juice, 30 ml (2 tbsp) water, 15 ml (1 tbsp) Italian seasoning and 15 ml (1 tbsp) whole-grain mustard. Add 1 can (398 ml) artichoke bottoms, drained and thinly sliced, 500 ml (2 cups) mâche and ½ head curly green lettuce, shredded. Toss.

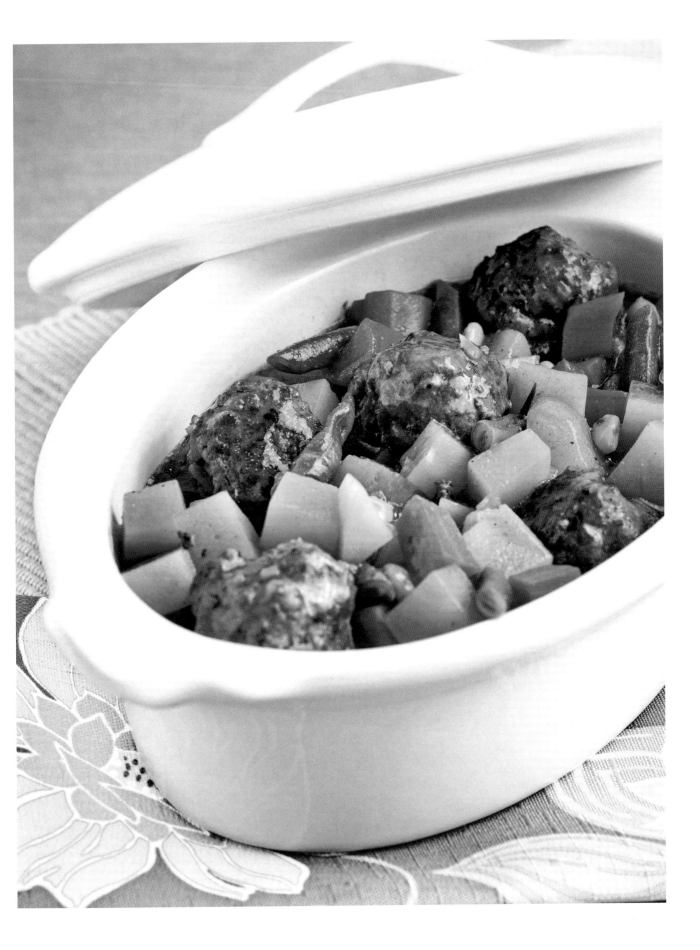

Satisfying Salads

A salad for dinner? Why not? Featuring a lovely mix of vegetables, fruits, grains, meat, fish, tofu, nuts or seafood, these salad recipes are loaded with vitamins, colours and flavours.

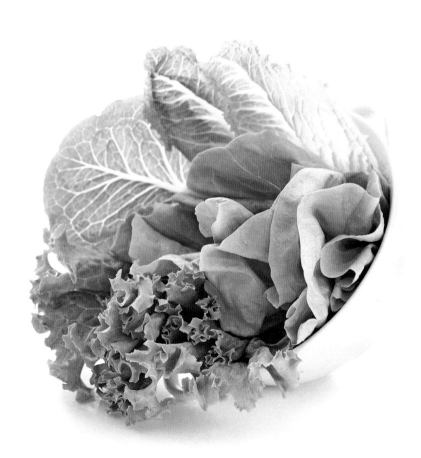

Teriyaki Chicken and Orange Salad

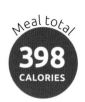

Meal total
398
CALORIES

4 skinless chicken breasts

15 ml (1 tbsp) sesame oil (untoasted)

For the marinade:

60 ml (¼ cup) soy sauce (low-sodium)

15 ml (1 tbsp) sesame oil (untoasted)

15 ml (1 tbsp) mirin

15 ml (1 tbsp) ginger, minced

10 ml (2 tsp) garlic, minced

For the vinaigrette:

30 ml (2 tbsp) canola oil

30 ml (2 tbsp) fresh cilantro, chopped

30 ml (2 tbsp) lime juice

30 ml (2 tbsp) lemon juice

15 ml (1 tbsp) honey

5 ml (1 tsp) garlic, minced

For the salad:

2 oranges

1 head green curly leaf lettuce, shredded

Prep time **30 minutes**

Marination **30 minutes**

Cook time **10 minutes**

Serves **4**

PER SERVING	
Calories	398
Protein	37 g
Fat	18 g
Carbohydrates	23 g
Fibre	4 g
Iron	2 mg
Calcium	108 mg
Sodium	700 mg

1. Mix all the marinade ingredients in an airtight bag. Add the chicken breasts to the bag and shake it. Let marinate in the refrigerator for 30 minutes to 1 hour.

2. While the chicken marinates, prepare the vinaigrette by whisking together all the ingredients in a bowl. Set aside in a cool place.

3. Supreme the oranges by using a knife to cut off the rind and then slicing along either side of the membranes. Remove the segments and set aside in a cool place.

4. When ready to cook, drain the chicken breasts and throw out the marinade. Heat the sesame oil in a frying pan over medium heat. Cook the breasts for 5 to 6 minutes on each side, until the meat is no longer pink in the centre. Place the breasts on a cutting board and let cool.

5. In a salad bowl, toss the lettuce with the vinaigrette. Add the orange supremes. Serve the salad onto plates.

6. Slice the breasts and place on the salad.

Did you know?

Oranges: Champions of vitamin C

Did you know that one orange packs all the vitamin C you need for a day? Even when compared to other citrus fruits, oranges stand out because of their exceptional vitamin C—and therefore antioxidant—content. Eating a single orange every day helps your body fight off oxidative stress, which is thought to be responsible for heart disease and cancer. Vitamin C also helps your body absorb the iron in vegetable-based foods, protects against infections and speeds up your body's scarring process.

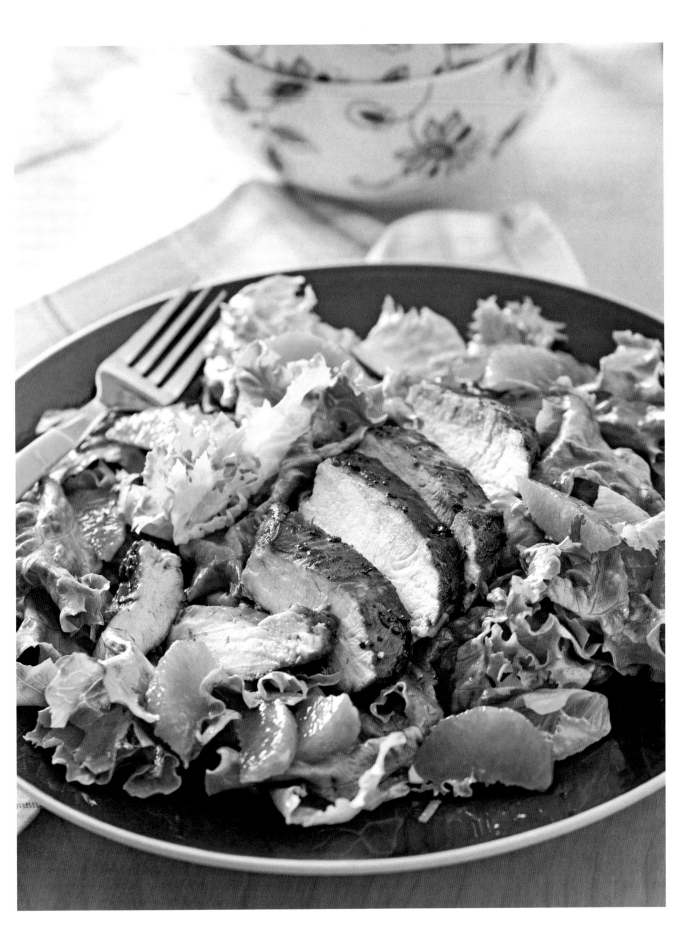

Chicken and Shrimp Salad

Meal total
356
CALORIES

For the dressing:

125 ml (½ cup) coconut milk

30 ml (2 tbsp) lime juice

15 ml (1 tbsp) ginger, minced

15 ml (1 tbsp) honey

10 ml (2 tsp) garlic, minced

5 ml (1 tsp) hot pepper, chopped (optional)

For the salad:

4 baby bok choy heads

1 celery stalk

1 red pepper

500 ml (2 cups) cooked chicken, sliced

250 ml (1 cup) northern shrimp

250 ml (1 cup) bean sprouts

60 ml (¼ cup) cilantro leaves

3 green onions, chopped

½ head romaine lettuce, shredded

Prep time **25 minutes**

Serves **4**

1. In a salad bowl, mix the dressing ingredients.

2. Chop the baby bok choy, celery and pepper.

3. Add the chopped vegetables and the rest of the ingredients to the salad bowl. Toss.

PER SERVING	
Calories	356
Protein	47 g
Fat	9 g
Carbohydrates	32 g
Fibre	12 g
Iron	10 mg
Calcium	961 mg
Sodium	878 mg

Did you know?

Coconut milk comes in light version!
If you're watching your figure, you might hesitate to cook with coconut milk because of its high saturated fat content. However, you should know that most stores now carry the light version. With 50% less fat, there are about 150 calories per 200 ml, depending on the brand.

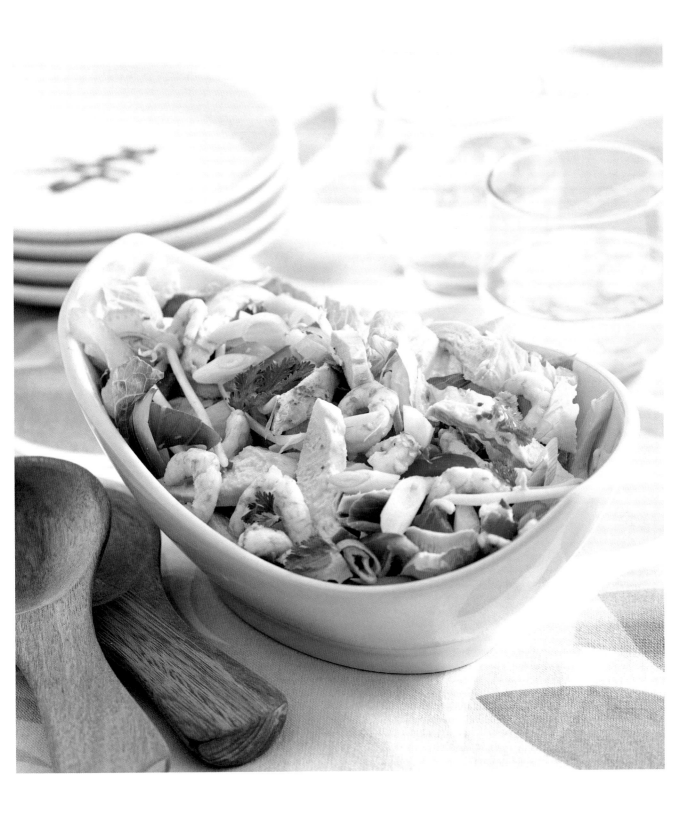

Tomato and Bocconcini Rice Salad

Meal total
343
CALORIES

250 ml (1 cup) rice

30 ml (2 tbsp) olive oil

30 ml (2 tbsp) lemon juice

30 ml (2 tbsp) vegetable stock

45 ml (3 tbsp) fresh mint, chopped

Salt and pepper to taste

16 cherry tomatoes, cut in half

½ container (200 g) bocconcini pearls

1 red onion, chopped

Prep time **15 minutes**

Cook time **15 minutes**

Serves **4**

PER SERVING	
Calories	343
Protein	9 g
Fat	13 g
Carbohydrates	47 g
Fibre	3 g
Iron	1 mg
Calcium	87 mg
Sodium	27 mg

1. Cook the rice according to the instruction on the packaging. Remove from the heat and let cool.

2. In a salad bowl, whisk together the oil, lemon juice, vegetable stock and mint. Season with salt and pepper.

3. Add the cherry tomatoes, bocconcini pearls, red onion and rice. Stir.

Did you know?

How to add a little extra protein

To ensure that your body functions properly (and that you can make it until the next meal!), you should eat meals that provide at least 15 g of protein. You can boost the protein levels in this delicious salad by adding any of the following ingredients to it.

PROTEIN SOURCE	QUANTITY	CALORIES	PROTEIN
Cooked chicken	60 ml (¼ cup)	+ 54 (total: 395)	+ 11 g (total: 20 g)
Tuna	60 ml (¼ cup)	+ 45 (total: 386)	+ 10 g (total: 19 g)
Lentils	80 ml (⅓ cup)	+ 78 (total: 419)	+ 6 g (total: 15 g)
Hard-boiled egg	1 egg	+ 71 (total: 412)	+ 6 g (total: 15 g)

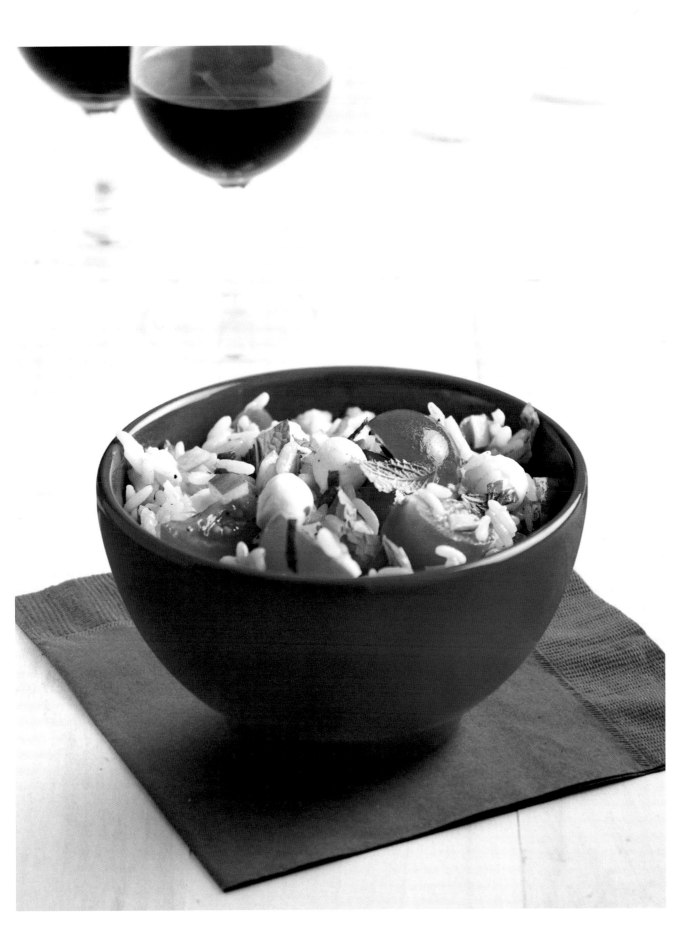

Edamame and Feta Quinoa Salad

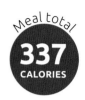

Meal total
337
CALORIES

180 ml (¾ cup) quinoa

180 ml (¾ cup) edamame

½ cucumber

1 yellow pepper

8 radishes

16 cherry tomatoes

30 ml (2 tbsp) olive oil

30 ml (2 tbsp) vegetable stock

45 ml (3 tbsp) fresh chives, chopped

30 ml (2 tbsp) fresh mint, chopped

30 ml (2 tbsp) lemon juice

Salt and pepper to taste

150 g plain or sun-dried tomato feta, diced

Prep time **15 minutes**

Cook time **20 minutes**

Serves **4**

PER SERVING	
Calories	337
Protein	14 g
Fat	18 g
Carbohydrates	32 g
Fibre	5 g
Iron	3 mg
Calcium	241 mg
Sodium	378 mg

1. Cook the quinoa according to the instructions on the packaging (about 20 minutes).

2. While the quinoa is cooking, cook the edamame in boiling, salted water for 5 minutes. Drain.

3. Dice the cucumber, pepper and radishes. Cut the tomatoes in half.

4. In a salad bowl, mix the oil with the vegetable stock, herbs and lemon juice. Season.

5. Add the vegetables, feta, quinoa and edamame. Toss.

Try it because...

Quinoa is a protein-rich grain

Originally from South America, quinoa is incredibly rich in iron and stands out because of its high levels of protein, vitamins, minerals and fibre. For example, 125 ml (½ cup) of quinoa contains as much fibre as a slice of whole wheat bread or 125 ml (½ cup) of cooked brown rice. Quinoa is delicious in salads, but it can also be added to soups or replace rice as a side. You can find quinoa in the natural food section at the supermarket.

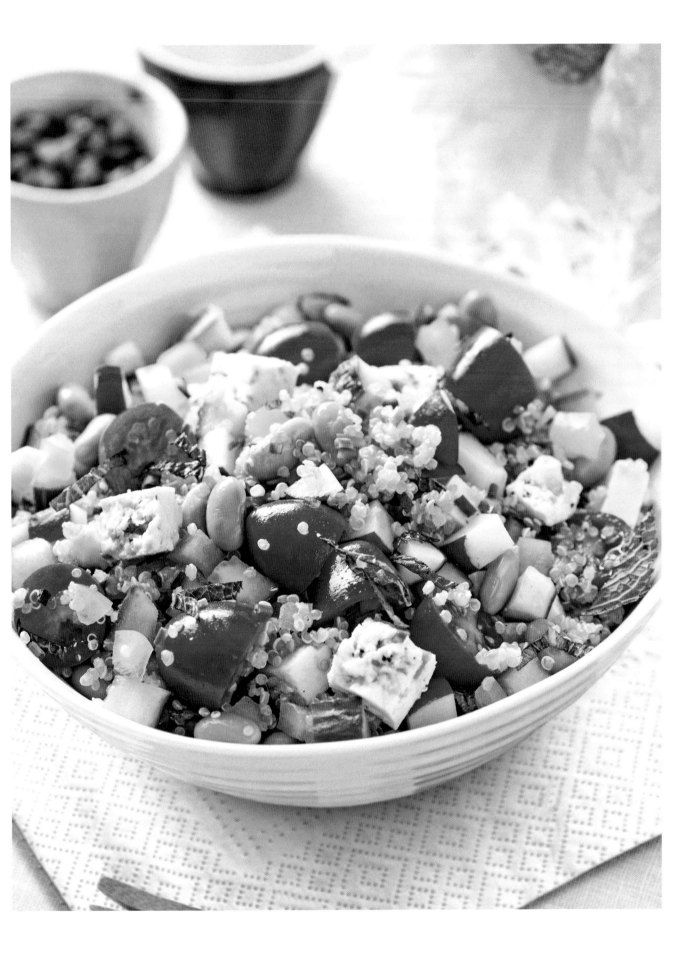

Chicken Caesar Salad

Meal total **340** CALORIES

¼ ciabatta baguette

2 slices prosciutto

1 head romaine lettuce, shredded

450 g (1 lb) grilled chicken, cut into strips

125 ml (½ cup) light mozzarella, shredded

30 ml (2 tbsp) fresh parsley, chopped

For the dressing:

90 ml (6 tbsp) plain yogourt (0%)

45 ml (3 tbsp) Parmesan, grated

15 ml (1 tbsp) milk

10 ml (2 tsp) garlic, minced

10 ml (2 tsp) lemon juice

10 ml (2 tsp) capers, chopped

Salt and pepper to taste

Prep time **15 minutes**

Cook time **8 minutes**

Serves **4**

PER SERVING	
Calories	340
Protein	47 g
Fat	9 g
Carbohydrates	15 g
Fibre	2 g
Iron	3 mg
Calcium	249 mg
Sodium	737 mg

1. Preheat the oven to 180°C (350°F).

2. Cut the baguette into small cubes. Place on a baking sheet lined with parchment paper. Bake for 8 to 10 minutes.

3. Place the prosciutto slices on another baking sheet lined with parchment paper. Bake for 8 to 10 minutes, until the prosciutto is golden-brown and crispy. Remove the baking sheet from the oven and break the prosciutto into pieces.

4. In a salad bowl, whisk together the dressing ingredients.

5. Add the romaine lettuce, prosciutto, chicken, mozzarella and parsley. Toss.

6. Serve the salad on plates. Top with croutons.

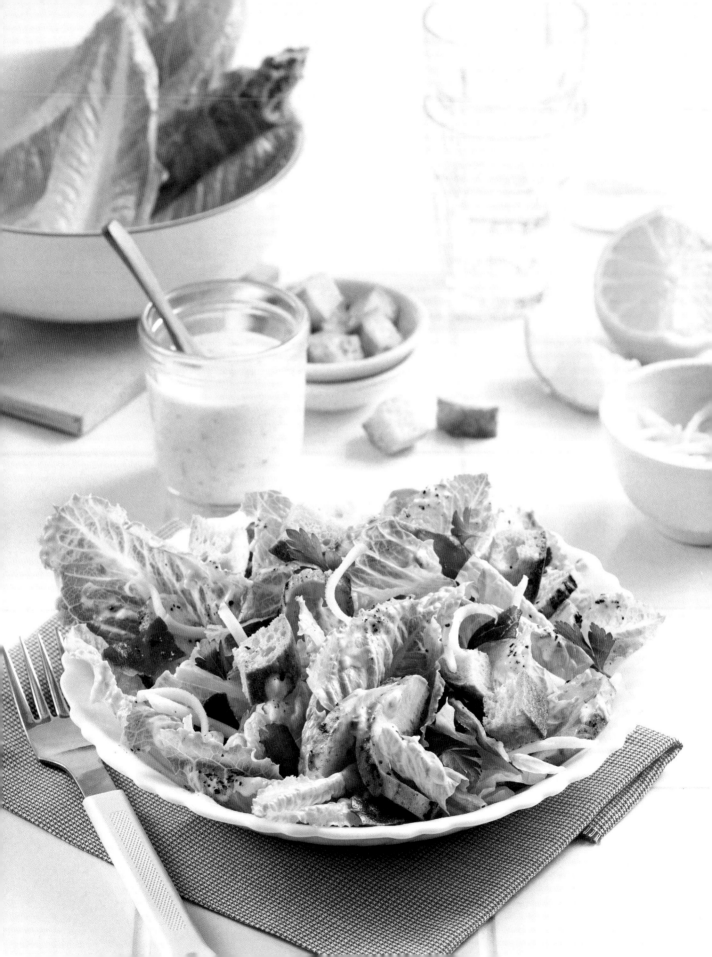

Potato and Smoked Salmon Salad

For the dressing:

45 ml (3 tbsp) light sour cream (4%)

45 ml (3 tbsp) plain Greek yogourt (0%)

1 lemon (juice)

Salt and pepper to taste

A few leaves parsley, chopped

For the salad:

8 whole creamer potatoes

1 cucumber

125 ml (½ cup) radishes, thinly sliced

30 ml (2 tbsp) fresh dill, chopped

1 package (225 g) smoked salmon

1 drizzle olive oil

Fleur de sel, to taste

Prep time **25 minutes**

Cook time **20 minutes**

Serves **4**

PER SERVING	
Calories	287
Protein	24 g
Fat	8 g
Carbohydrates	31 g
Fibre	5 g
Iron	1 mg
Calcium	81 mg
Sodium	449 mg

1. Cook the potatoes al dente in a pot of boiling, salted water for 20 minutes. Drain and let cool.

2. In a salad bowl, whisk together all the dressing ingredients.

3. Peel and remove the seeds from the cucumber. Use a peeler to slice it lengthwise into long strips. Slice the potatoes.

4. Add the cucumber strips, radishes and dill to the salad bowl. Gently mix.

5. Arrange a rosette of overlapping potato slices on a plate. Top with the vegetable salad and slices of smoked salmon. Drizzle with olive oil and sprinkle with fleur de sel.

Try it because...

Smoked salmon is good for you!

Salmon is a healthy food source for multiple reasons. Whether fresh or smoked, this fish is an excellent source of omega-3 fatty acids and helps meet your requirement of vitamins B12 and D. Plus, its high level of protein means you'll be left feeling satisfied and satiated. Smoked salmon, however, does have higher levels of sodium and fat than the fresh version. A 75 g serving of smoked salmon has an average of 225 mg of sodium, 5 g of fat and 23 g of protein. The same quantity of fresh salmon contains 64 mg of sodium, 3 g of fat and 19 g of protein.

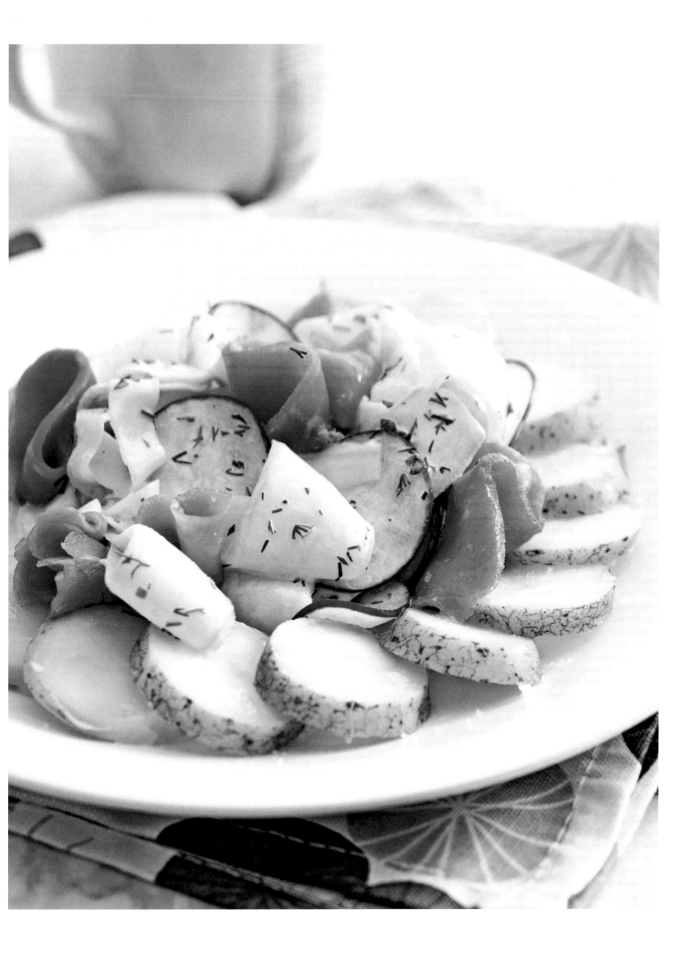

Poached Salmon and Apple Salad

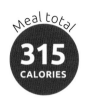

Meal total
315
CALORIES

For the salmon:

1 litre (4 cups) water

½ onion, chopped

5 peppercorns

1 bay leaf

1 large pinch salt

1 celery stalk

500 g (about 1 lb) skinless salmon fillets

For the salad:

375 ml (1 ½ cups) cauliflower, cut into small florets

1 head iceberg lettuce, shredded

1 green apple, diced

15 ml (1 tbsp) fresh dill, chopped

For the vinaigrette:

45 ml (3 tbsp) olive oil

30 ml (2 tbsp) lemon juice

15 ml (1 tbsp) orange juice

Salt to taste

Prep time **20 minutes**

Cook time **5 minutes**

Serves **4**

1. Place the water, onion, peppercorns, bay leaf, salt and celery in a pot and bring to a boil.

2. Add the salmon fillets. Cover and cook for over low heat for 5 minutes. Remove the fillets and place on paper towels.

3. Cook the cauliflower in a pot of boiling water for 5 minutes, until tender. Rinse under cold water and drain.

4. In a salad bowl, mix the vinaigrette ingredients.

5. Add the lettuce, apple, dill and cauliflower to the bowl. Toss.

6. Serve the salad onto plates. Top with the salmon.

PER SERVING	
Calories	315
Protein	28 g
Fat	19 g
Carbohydrates	15 g
Fibre	4 g
Iron	2 mg
Calcium	80 mg
Sodium	194 mg

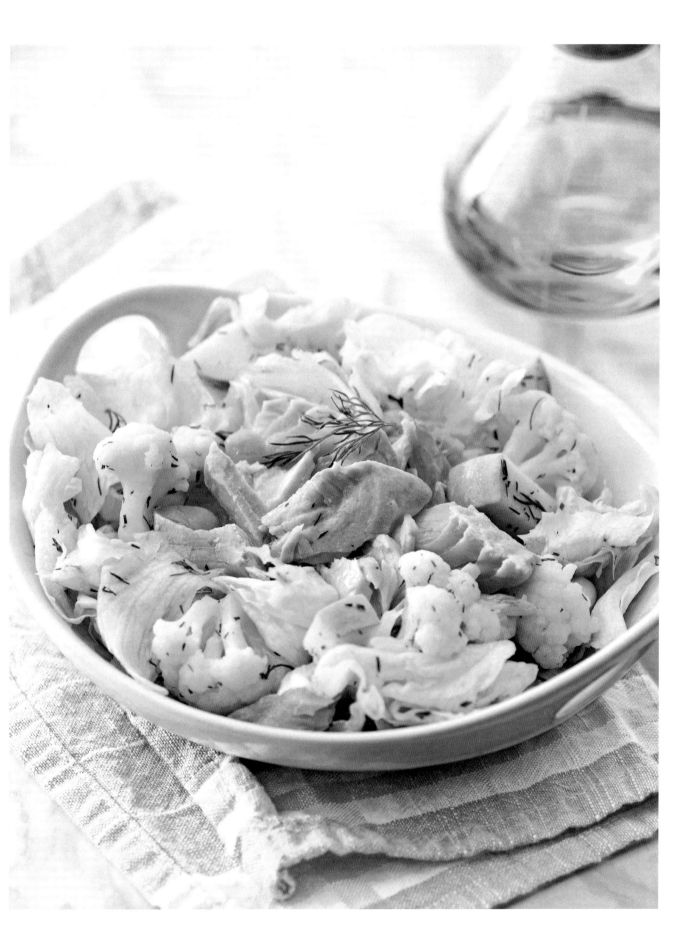

Tuna Salade Niçoise

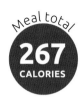

4 eggs

150 g (⅓ lb) green and yellow beans

2 cans (170 g each) tuna, drained

2 Italian tomatoes, cut into wedges

1 litre (4 cups) romaine lettuce, shredded

1 small red onion, thinly sliced

30 ml (2 tbsp) fresh basil, chopped

125 ml (½ cup) Greek vinaigrette

Salt and pepper to taste

Prep time **15 minutes**

Cook time **10 minutes**

Serves **4**

PER SERVING	
Calories	267
Protein	30 g
Fat	12 g
Carbohydrates	11 g
Fibre	3 g
Iron	3 mg
Calcium	76 mg
Sodium	508 mg

1. Place the eggs in a pot and cover with cold water. Bring to a boil and cook for 10 minutes over medium heat. Drain and submerge in ice water. Peel the eggs and then cut into wedges.

2. While the eggs are cooking, place the beans in another pot of boiling, salted water. Bring to a boil and cook for 5 minutes. Drain and submerge in ice water.

3. Gently mix all the ingredients together in a salad bowl.

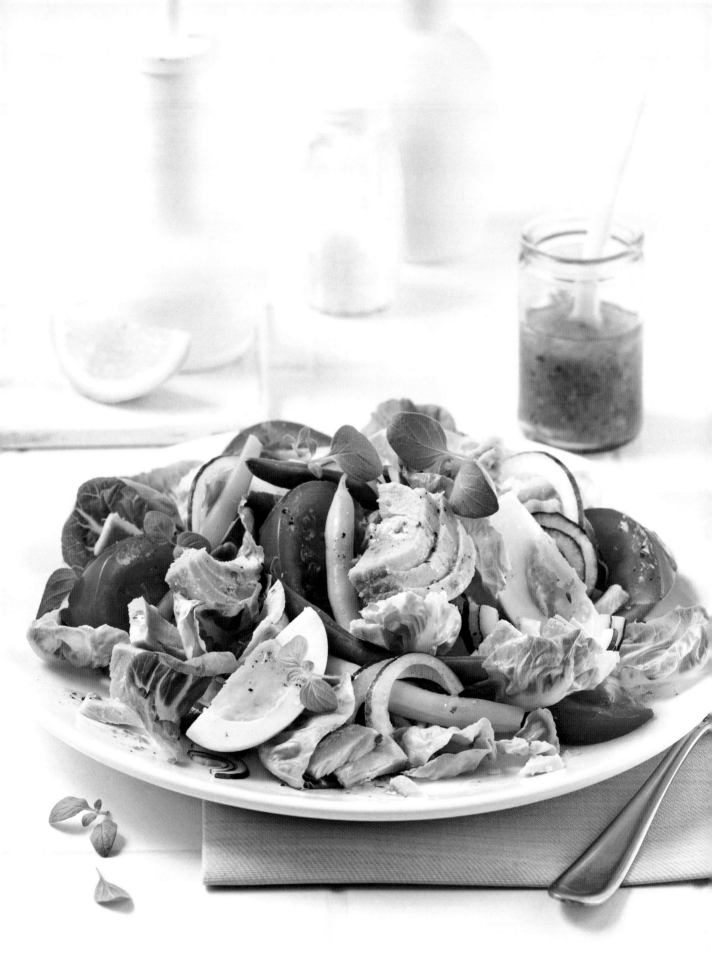

Warm Chicken Couscous Salad

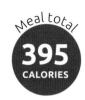

Meal total
395
CALORIES

250 ml (1 cup) couscous

30 ml (2 tbsp) olive oil

Salt and pepper to taste

250 ml (1 cup) boiling water

3 skinless chicken breasts

1 English cucumber

1 yellow pepper

16 cherry tomatoes

30 ml (2 tbsp) lemon juice

A few mint leaves, chopped

Prep time **15 minutes**

Cook time **3 minutes**

Serves **4**

PER SERVING	
Calories	395
Protein	32 g
Fat	10 g
Carbohydrates	44 g
Fibre	4 g
Iron	2 mg
Calcium	41 mg
Sodium	60 mg

1. In a large bowl, mix the couscous with 15 ml (1 tbsp) of oil. Season with salt and pepper. Add the boiling water. Cover and let the couscous steam for 5 minutes.

2. Dice the chicken breasts. Heat the rest of the oil in a frying pan over medium heat. Brown the chicken for 3 to 4 minutes, until the meat is no longer pink in the centre. Remove from the heat and set aside.

3. Dice the cucumber and pepper. Slice the tomatoes in half.

4. Fluff the couscous with a fork. Add the vegetables, chicken, lemon juice and mint.

Did you know?

We eat too much salt!
Always go for recipes or products that are considered low in sodium, meaning they contain no more than 140 mg of sodium. Health Canada recommends consuming between 1,000 and 1,500 mg of sodium a day. However, most people consume about 3,600 mg a day, or more than double the daily recommended value. Cooking with whole foods and avoiding processed foods as much as possible—like store-bought sauces or dressings—are definitely the best ways to reduce your salt intake.

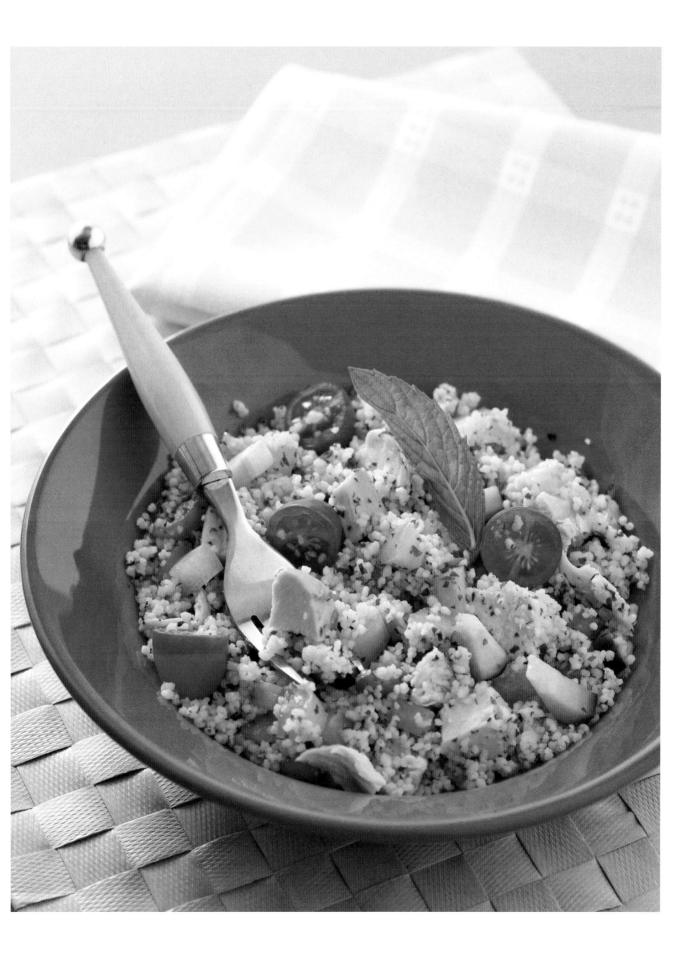

Greek Salad

1 cucumber

4 large tomatoes

1 green pepper

½ red onion

30 ml (2 tbsp) water

16 Kalamata olives

30 ml (2 tbsp) olive oil

1 container (200 g) feta

5 ml (1 tsp) dried oregano

Pepper to taste

Prep time **15 minutes**

Serves **4**

PER SERVING	
Calories	286
Protein	10 g
Fat	21 g
Carbohydrates	17 g
Fibre	4 g
Iron	1 mg
Calcium	291 mg
Sodium	765 mg

1. Chop the cucumber and cut the tomatoes into wedges. Thinly slice the pepper and red onion.

2. In a salad bowl, mix the vegetables with the water, olives and half of the olive oil.

3. Cut the feta into four slices.

4. Serve the salad on plates. Top each serving with a slice of feta. Sprinkle with oregano and drizzle with the rest of the olive oil. Season with pepper.

Try it with...
Cheesy Pita Wedges
Per serving: 110 calories
In a bowl, mix 10 ml (2 tsp) olive oil with 15 ml (1 tbsp) Greek seasoning, 15 ml (1 tbsp) lemon zest and 45 ml (3 tbsp) shredded Romano cheese (or mozzarella). Brush 3 pitas with the flavoured oil. Cut each pita into eight wedges. Place the pita wedges on a baking sheet lined with parchment paper. Bake for 8 to 10 minutes at 190°C (375°F).

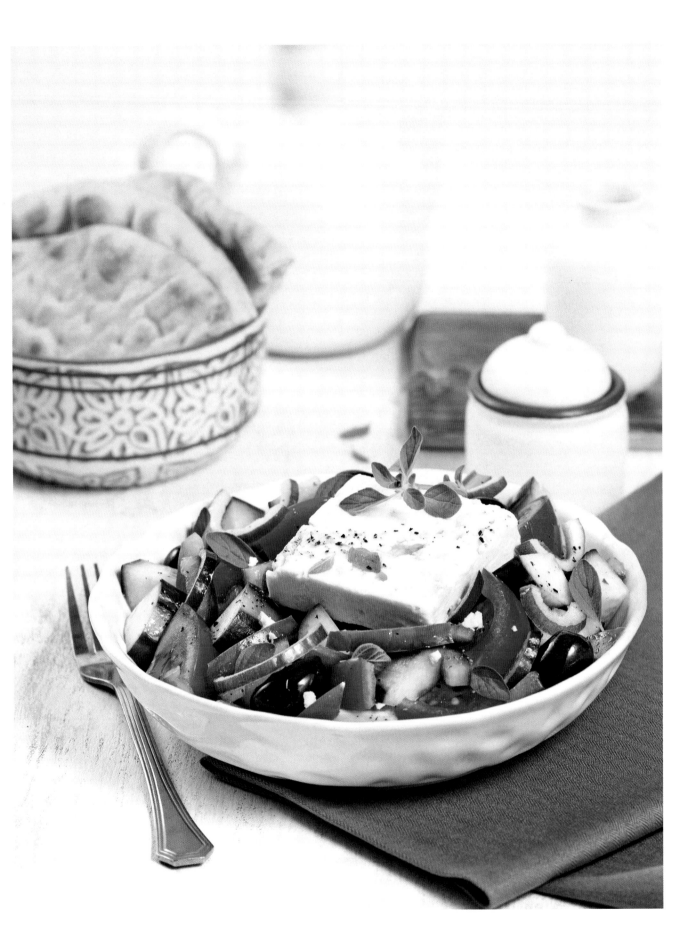

Pizza & pasta

Whether it's for lunch or dinner, it's always a good time when pizza or pasta is on the menu! Great for any occasion, these two dishes combine flavours and colours to create a happy feast that looks as good as it tastes.

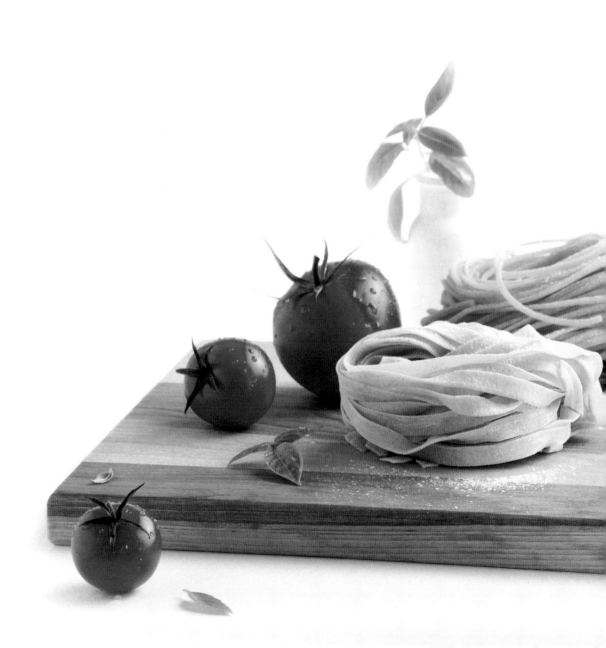

Grilled Vegetable Pizza

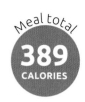

Meal total
389
CALORIES

2 medium zucchinis

1 medium eggplant

Salt and pepper
to taste

1 thin pizza crust (250 g)

125 ml (½ cup)
strained tomatoes

180 ml (¾ cup)
mozzarella, shredded

125 ml (½ cup)
Parmesan, grated

Prep time **20 minutes**

Cook time **10 minutes**

Serves **4**

PER SERVING	
Calories	337
Protein	15 g
Fat	11 g
Carbohydrates	47 g
Fibre	7 g
Iron	3 mg
Calcium	260 mg
Sodium	769 mg

1. Preheat the oven to 230°C (450°F).

2. Use a peeler to cut the zucchinis into long strips and the eggplant into thin slices.

3. Cook the vegetables in a non-stick grill pan for about 1 minute on each side. Remove from the pan and set aside on a plate. Season with salt and pepper.

4. Place the pizza crust on a baking sheet. Spread the strained tomatoes onto the crust. Lightly season with salt and pepper. Arrange the vegetables in a rosette around the crust. Sprinkle with the mozzarella and Parmesan.

5. Bake for 10 minutes, until the crust is golden-brown and the cheese is melted.

Try it with...

Arugula Salad
Per serving: 52 calories
Mix 3 Italian tomatoes, diced, with 10 ml (2 tsp) olive oil and 500 ml (2 cups) arugula. Season with salt and pepper. Add 45 ml (3 tbsp) Parmesan shavings and a few leaves of basil.

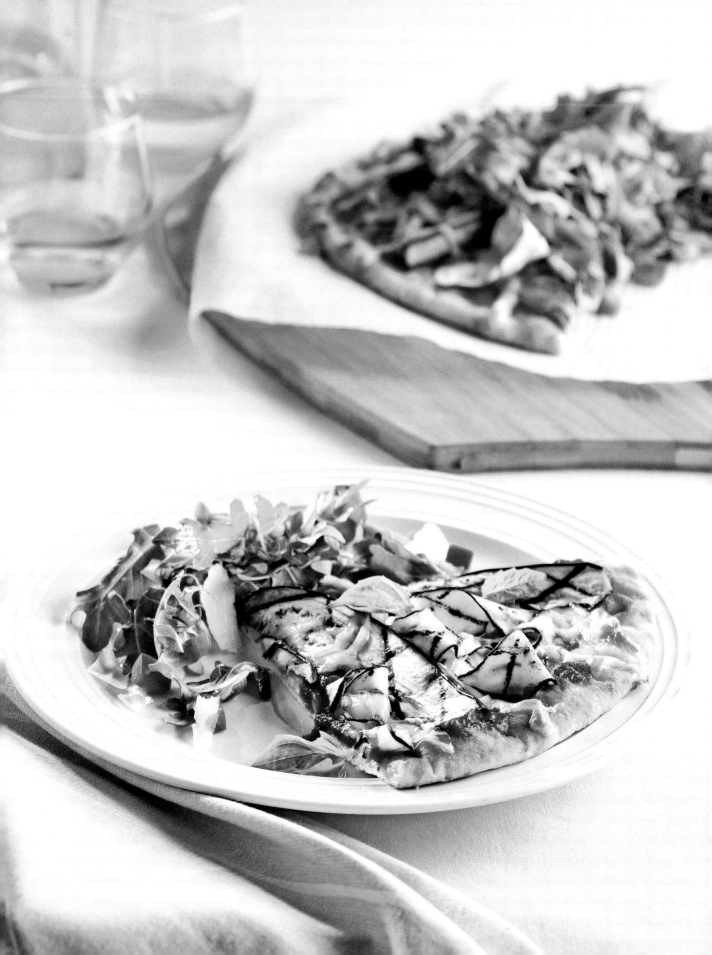

Ham Lasagna

4 lasagna sheets

45 ml (3 tbsp) olive oil

1 onion, diced

500 ml (2 cups) ham, diced

1 zucchini, diced

16 grape tomatoes, cut in half

250 ml (1 cup) arugula

30 ml (2 tbsp) basil pesto

80 ml (⅓ cup) Parmesan, grated

Prep time **15 minutes**

Cook time **10 minutes**

Serves **4**

PER SERVING	
Calories	355
Protein	18 g
Fat	20 g
Carbohydrates	26 g
Fibre	2 g
Iron	2 mg
Calcium	99 mg
Sodium	1,075 mg

1. Cook the lasagna sheets *al dente* in a pot of boiling, salted water. Drain and leave in the pot with the lid on.

2. Heat 15 ml (1 tbsp) of olive oil in a frying pan over medium heat. Cook the onion, ham and zucchini for 2 minutes. Add the tomatoes and arugula. Cook for 1 minute.

3. In a small bowl, mix the pesto with the rest of the oil.

4. Place one lasagna sheet in each plate. Spread a third of the pesto onto the base of each lasagna sheet and then cover with a third of the ham mixture. Fold the noodles onto the mixture to form a second layer. Repeat twice and top with Parmesan.

Did you know?

Arugula is nutritious!

Arugula is a vegetable in the cruciferous family, along with broccoli and cabbage. It's low in calories and contains a healthy dose of vitamins K and B9 (folic acid). It also contains calcium, which is rather rare for a vegetable. But the main attraction is its abundance of flavonoids and carotenoids—antioxidants that could prevent and slow the progression of some types of cancer. Arugula leaves are slightly spicy, almost like mustard, and are frequently used in salads. Choose small leaves that are fresh, tender and narrow.

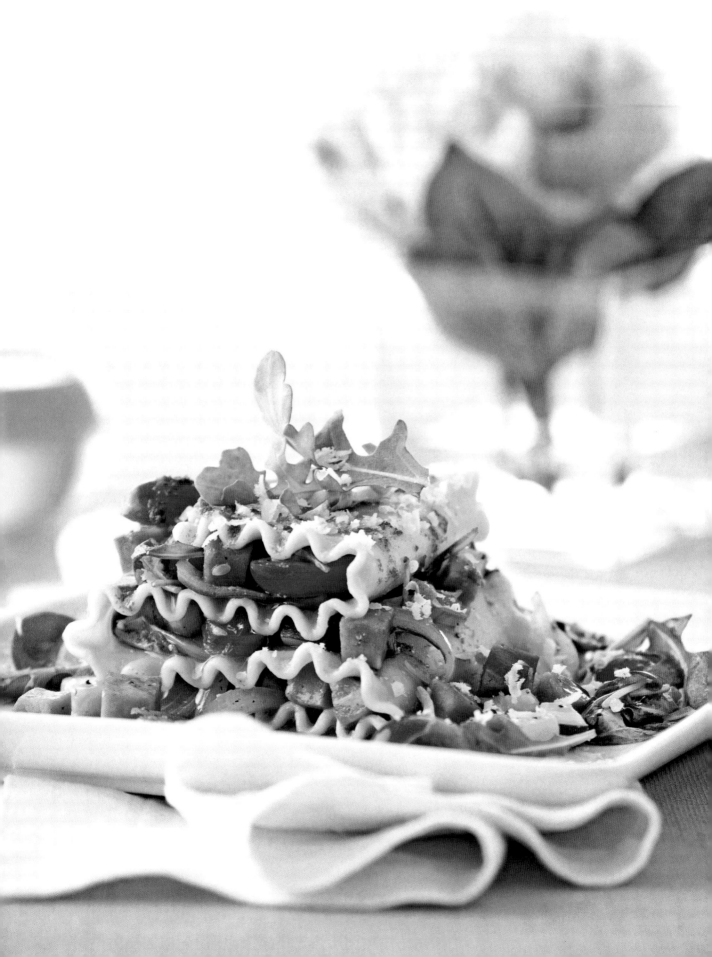

Cherry Tomato and Pine Nut Spaghetti

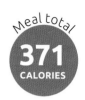

Meal total
371
CALORIES

250 g spaghetti noodles

30 ml (2 tbsp) olive oil

1 onion, chopped

45 ml (3 tbsp) pine nuts

10 ml (2 tsp) garlic, minced

16 cherry tomatoes, cut in half

Salt and pepper to taste

A few basil leaves

45 ml (3 tbsp) Parmesan, grated

Parmesan shavings (optional)

Prep time **15 minutes**

Cook time **10 minutes**

Serves **4**

PER SERVING	
Calories	371
Protein	11 g
Fat	14 g
Carbohydrates	52 g
Fibre	3 g
Iron	3 mg
Calcium	67 mg
Sodium	94 mg

1. Cook the pasta *al dente* in a pot of boiling, salted water. Drain.

2. Heat the oil in another pot over medium heat. Brown the onion for 2 minutes. Add the pine nuts, garlic and cherry tomatoes. Cook for 2 minutes.

3. Add the pasta and the rest of the ingredients.

4. Sprinkle each serving with Parmesan shavings if desired.

Did you know?

What are the nutritional qualities of tomatoes?

Juicy, nutritious and refreshing, tomatoes have come to play an important role in our diet. Low in calories, this fruit has a high water content (91%) and is a good source of vitamin C and potassium. It also contains folic acid and vitamin A, and its high level of antioxidants (lycopene) gives it its bright red colour and even helps lower the risk of some cancers. Eaten either raw or cooked, tomatoes are one of the most versatile foods you could incorporate into your daily menu.

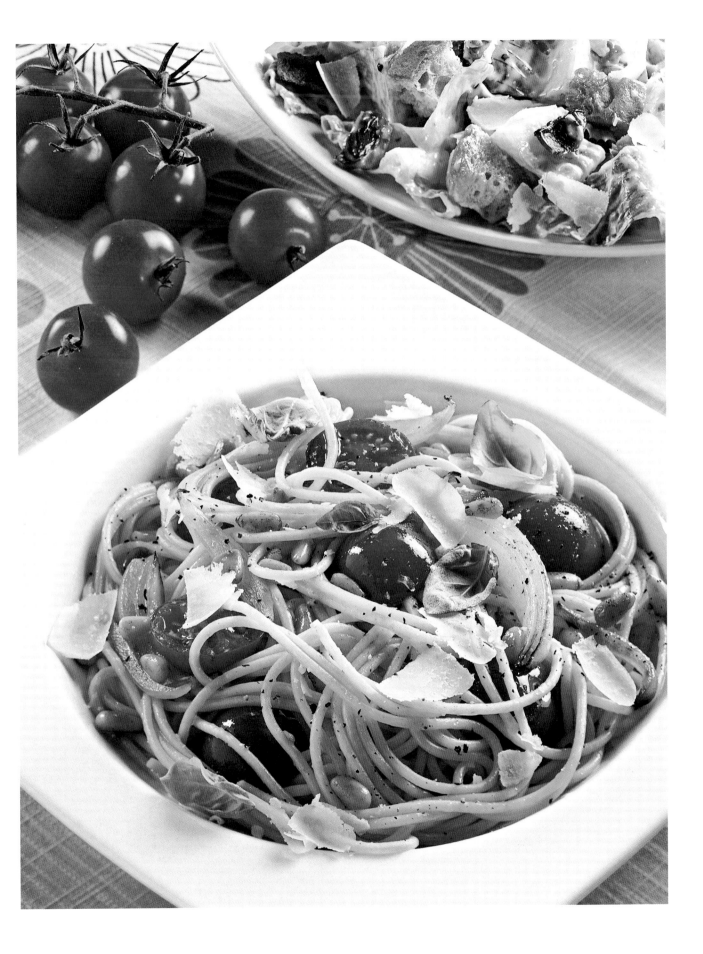

Mini Barbecue Chicken Pizzas

Meal total

388
CALORIES

125 ml (½ cup) barbecue sauce

375 ml (1 ½ cups) cooked chicken, chopped

4 tomatoes, diced

1 yellow pepper, diced

15 ml (1 tbsp) olive oil

5 ml (1 tsp) garlic, minced

30 ml (2 tbsp) fresh basil, chopped

Salt and pepper to taste

6 thin hamburger buns

1 red onion, thinly sliced

375 ml (1 ½ cups) mozzarella, shredded

Prep time **20 minutes**

Cook time **6 minutes**

Serves **6 (12 mini-pizzas)**

PER SERVING 2 mini-pizzas	
Calories	388
Protein	26 g
Fat	10 g
Carbohydrates	50 g
Fibre	2 g
Iron	2 mg
Calcium	306 mg
Sodium	663 mg

1. Preheat the oven to 205°C (400°F).

2. In a large bowl, mix half of the barbecue sauce with the chicken.

3. In another bowl, mix the tomatoes with the pepper, oil, garlic and basil. Season with salt and pepper.

4. Slice the buns in half and brush with the rest of the barbecue sauce. Place the buns on a baking sheet. Top with the tomato mixture, chicken, onion and mozzarella. Bake for 6 to 8 minutes.

Try it because...

Mini means convenient!

What do pita bread, ciabatta bread, English muffins and thin hamburger buns have in common? They can be topped with your favourite ingredients and transformed into delectable to-go pizzas! These mini pizzas can be eaten hot or cold and are easy to pack for lunch. They also freeze easily, so you can keep some around for days when you're feeling uninspired. Visit the bakery section at your supermarket to find more ideas for your mini pizza lunches.

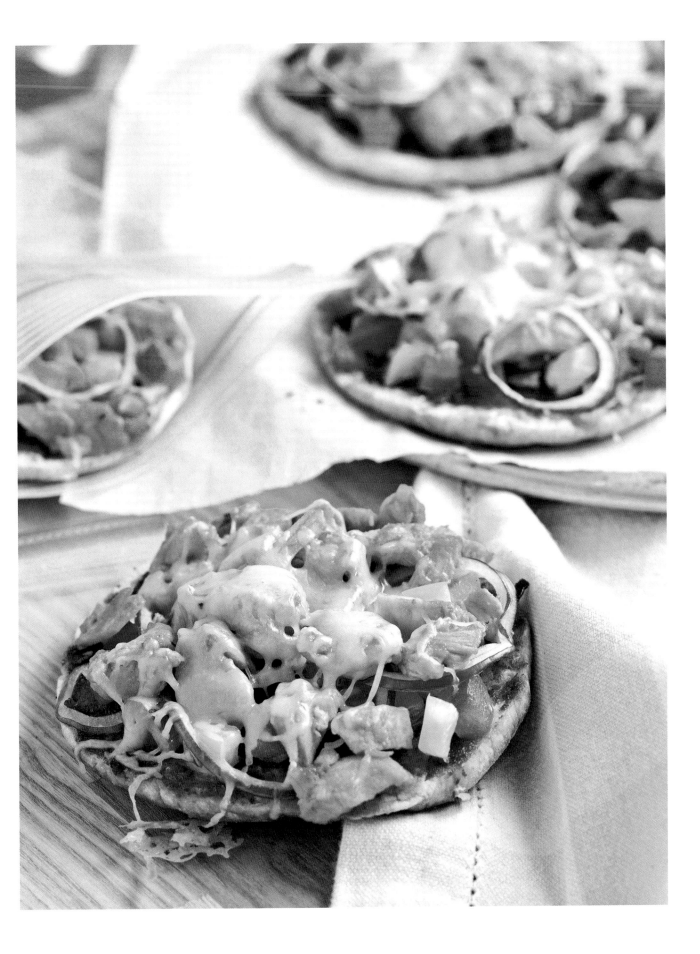

Chicken and Penne Cacciatore

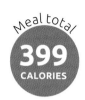

Meal total
399
CALORIES

225 g penne pasta

For the sauce:

30 ml (2 tbsp) olive oil

2 skinless chicken breasts, diced

1 onion, chopped

10 mushrooms, sliced

15 ml (1 tbsp) garlic, minced

80 ml (⅓ cup) white wine

250 ml (1 cup) chicken stock

1 can (540 ml) diced tomatoes

45 ml (3 tbsp) tomato paste

15 ml (1 tbsp) fresh oregano, chopped

15 ml (1 tbsp) brown sugar

1 bay leaf

Salt and pepper to taste

Prep time **25 minutes**

Cook time **21 minutes**

Serves **4**

PER SERVING	
Calories	399
Protein	27 g
Fat	7 g
Carbohydrates	54 g
Fibre	5 g
Iron	4 mg
Calcium	50 mg
Sodium	265 mg

1. Heat the oil in a pot over medium heat. Sear a few pieces of chicken at a time for 2 to 3 minutes, until the meat is golden-brown on all sides. Set aside the pieces of chicken on a plate.

2. In the pot, cook the onion, mushrooms and garlic for 1 minute over medium heat. Put the chicken back into the pot.

3. Pour in the wine and stock. Bring to a boil, scraping the browned bits from the sides of the pot with a wooden spoon. Add the rest of the ingredients. Cover and let simmer over medium-low heat for 18 to 20 minutes.

4. While the chicken is cooking, cook the pasta *al dente* in a pot of boiling, salted water. Drain.

5. Add the pasta to the pot and mix.

Did you know?

What is chicken cacciatore?
Chicken cacciatore (meaning "hunter-style" chicken) is an Italian dish that primarily consists of braised chicken, tomatoes, onions, mushrooms, various herbs and red or white wine. As is the case for most traditional dishes, there are several versions of this recipe. For example, some cooks add peppers, carrots, capers and olives.

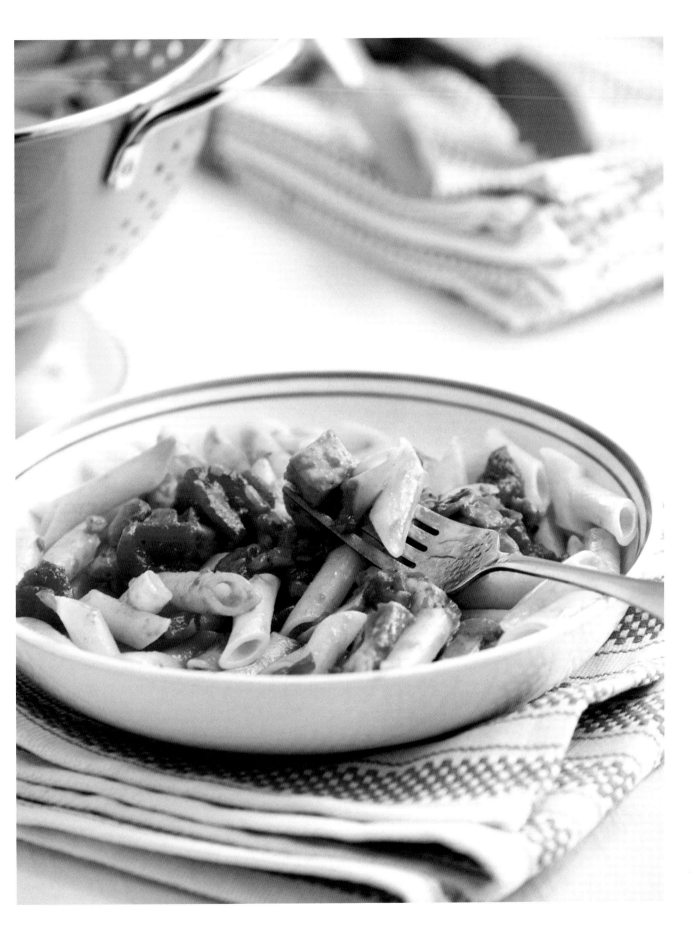

Chicken and Broccoli Farfalle

Meal total
391
CALORIES

225 g farfalle pasta

1 broccoli, cut into small florets

15 ml (1 tbsp) olive oil

2 skinless chicken breasts,
cut into strips

30 ml (2 tbsp) whole-grain
mustard

80 ml (⅓ cup) orange juice

Salt and pepper to taste

45 ml (3 tbsp) sliced almonds,
toasted

Prep time **15 minutes**

Cook time **5 minutes**

Serves **4**

PER SERVING	
Calories	391
Protein	27 g
Fat	11 g
Carbohydrates	48 g
Fibre	4 g
Iron	3 mg
Calcium	59 mg
Sodium	157 mg

1. Cook the pasta *al dente* in a pot of boiling, salted water. Add the broccoli to the pot 3 minutes before the pasta is done cooking. Drain.

2. Heat the oil in a large frying pan over medium heat. Brown the chicken strips for 2 to 3 minutes.

3. Add the mustard and orange juice to the pan and bring to a boil. Add the pasta and broccoli. Season with salt and pepper. Heat for another 1 to 2 minutes, stirring.

4. Sprinkle each serving with almonds.

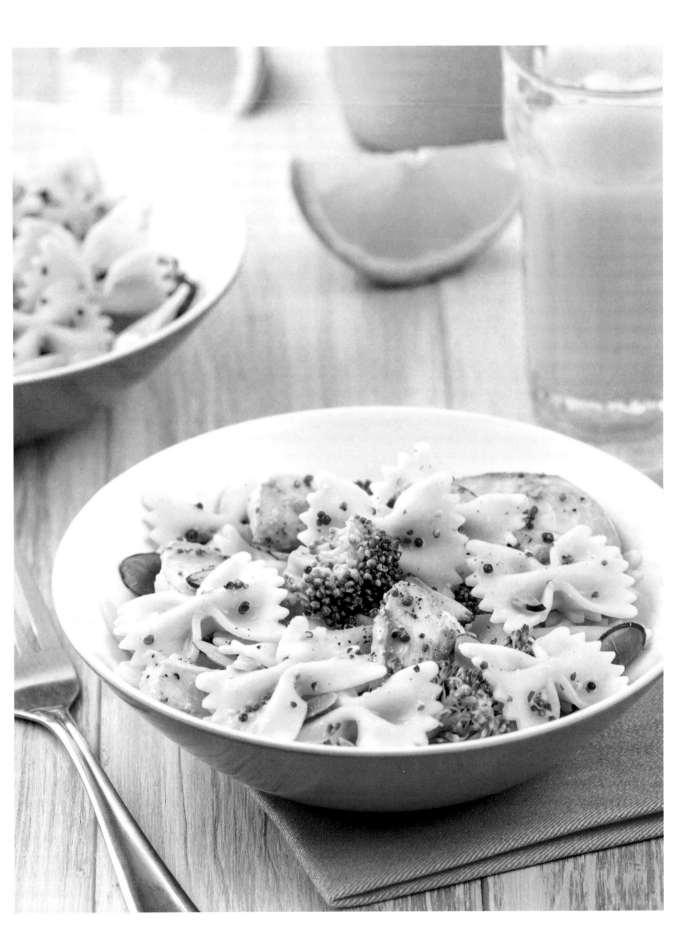

Shrimp and Pollock Capellini

Meal total
372
CALORIES

225 g capellini pasta

1 broccoli, cut into small florets

250 ml (1 cup) 1% milk

125 g light cream cheese

60 ml (¼ cup) fresh dill, chopped

250 ml (1 cup) northern shrimp

½ package (227 g) pollock, shredded

Salt and pepper to taste

Prep time **15 minutes**

Cook time **5 minutes**

Serves **4**

PER SERVING	
Calories	372
Protein	22 g
Fat	7 g
Carbohydrates	55 g
Fibre	3 g
Iron	1 mg
Calcium	158 mg
Sodium	550 mg

1. Cook the pasta with the broccoli in a pot of boiling, salted water for about 3 minutes. Drain.

2. Heat the milk and the cream cheese in the same pot over medium heat, whisking until it starts to simmer.

3. Add the dill, shrimp and pollock. Season with salt and pepper and cook for 2 minutes.

4. Add the pasta and broccoli. Stir and serve immediately.

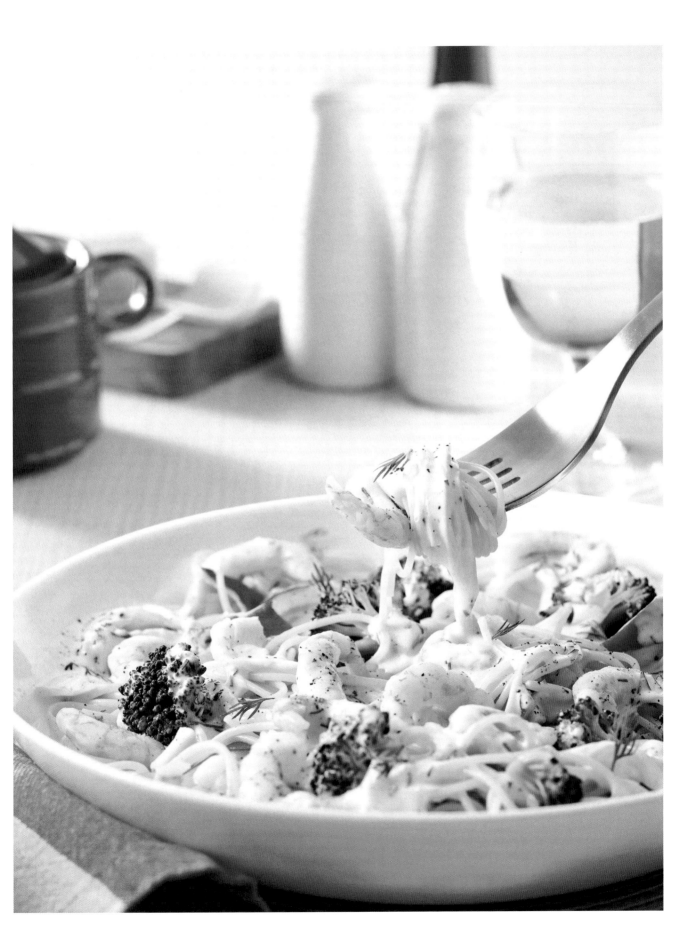

Spaghetti With Meat and Vegetable Sauce

Meal total
394
CALORIES

225 g spaghetti noodles

15 ml (1 tbsp) olive oil

225 g (about ½ lb) extra-lean ground beef

1 onion, chopped

375 ml (1 ½ cups) frozen diced vegetable mix

1 can (398 ml) tomato sauce

1 can (540 ml) diced tomatoes with Italian spices

Salt and pepper to taste

Prep time **15 minutes**

Cook time **15 minutes**

Serves **4**

PER SERVING	
Calories	394
Protein	22 g
Fat	9 g
Carbohydrates	57 g
Fibre	5 g
Iron	3 mg
Calcium	82 mg
Sodium	231 mg

1. Cook the pasta *al dente* in a pot of boiling, salted water. Drain.

2. While the pasta is cooking, heat the oil in another pot over medium heat. Cook the beef with the onion for 2 to 3 minutes, stirring so that the meat separates.

3. Add the vegetables. Add the tomato sauce and diced tomatoes. Season with salt and pepper. Let simmer, uncovered, for 15 minutes over medium heat. Serve with the pasta.

Did you know?

Does pasta cause weight gain?

From a nutritional standpoint, no single food alone has the ability to make you gain weight. However, pasta dishes *do* have a high calorie content. They contain an average of nearly 250 calories for every 250 ml (1 cup), so those who frequently enjoy pasta dishes will have to be more mindful of their serving sizes and pay closer attention to the seasonings and sauces that often come with them. You shouldn't have more than two servings per meal (125 ml—½ cup of cooked pasta equals one serving of grains), and choose whole grain pastas served with a sauce packed with vegetables to feel more satiated.

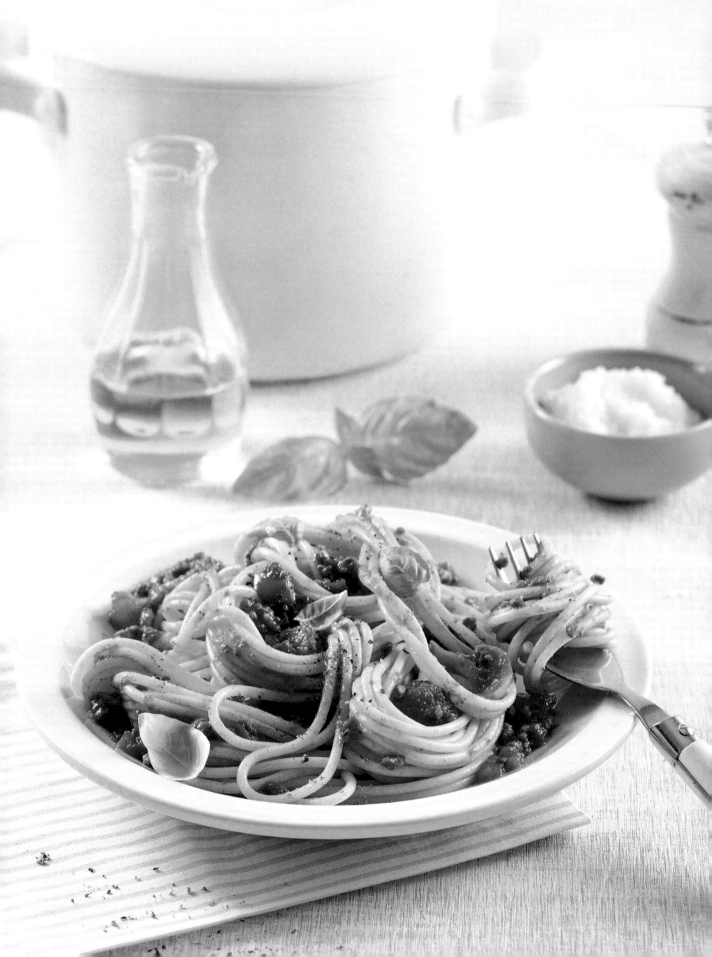

Cauliflower, Chickpea and Parmesan Penne

Meal total
384
CALORIES

240 g penne pasta

500 ml (2 cups) cauliflower,
cut into small florets

375 ml (1 ½ cups) chickpeas,
rinsed and drained

1 lemon (juice and zest)

A few leaves parsley, chopped

Salt and pepper to taste

125 ml (½ cup)
Parmesan, grated

Prep time **20 minutes**

Cook time **10 minutes**

Serves **4**

PER SERVING	
Calories	384
Protein	17 g
Fat	7 g
Carbohydrates	64 g
Fibre	8 g
Iron	4 mg
Calcium	166 mg
Sodium	560 mg

1. Cook the pasta *al dente* in a
large pot of boiling, salted water.
Add the cauliflower to the pot
5 minutes before the pasta is
done cooking. Drain, but keep
the cooking water.

2. Lightly crush the chickpeas with
a fork. Place them in the pot and
add 250 ml (1 cup) of the reserved
cooking water.

3. Add the pasta and the rest of the
ingredients, except the lemon zest.
Mix well and heat for 1 to 2 minutes.
If the mixture is too dry, add a little
more of the cooking water.

4. Sprinkle each serving with
lemon zest.

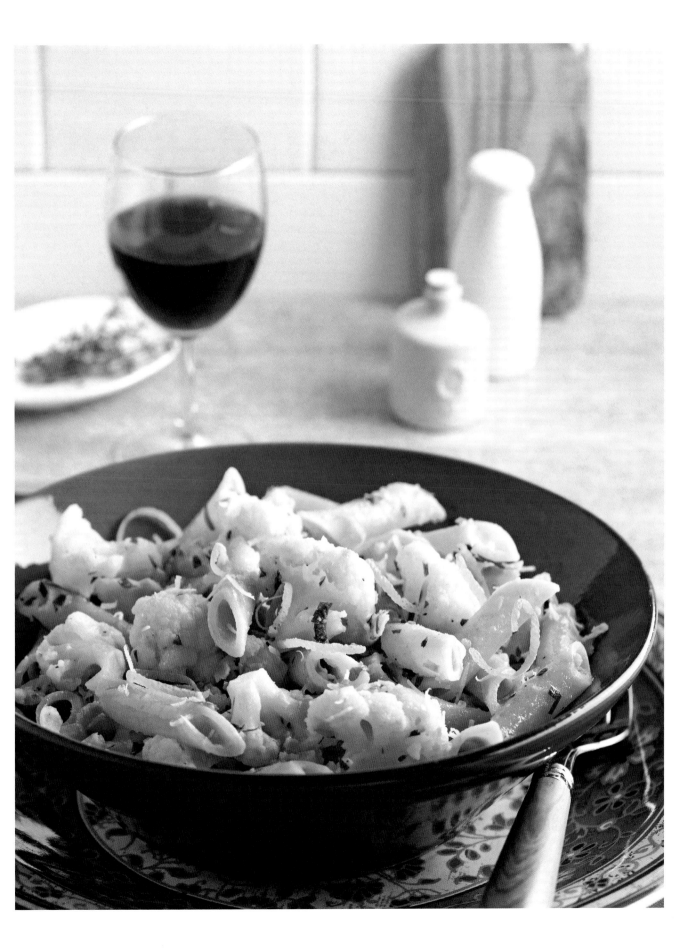

Tuna, Olive and Cherry Tomato Pasta

Meal total
388
CALORIES

225 g spaghetti noodles

7.5 ml (½ tbsp) olive oil

20 cherry tomatoes, cut in half

2 cans (120 g) white tuna,
drained and cut into pieces

20 Kalamata olives, cut in half

1 lemon (juice and zest)

Salt and pepper to taste

4 green onions, chopped

Prep time **15 minutes**

Cook time **10 minutes**

Serves **4**

PER SERVING	
Calories	388
Protein	29 g
Fat	8 g
Carbohydrates	49 g
Fibre	4 g
Iron	3 mg
Calcium	59 mg
Sodium	646 mg

1. Cook the pasta *al dente* in a pot of boiling, salted water. Drain, but keep 80 ml (⅓ cup) of the cooking water.

2. Heat the oil in a large frying pan over medium heat. Cook the tomatoes for about 1 minute, until they become slightly soft. Add the tuna, olives, and the lemon juice and zest. Season with salt and pepper.

3. Add the pasta and mix well. If the mixture is too dry, add the reserved cooking water.

4. Sprinkle each serving with green onions.

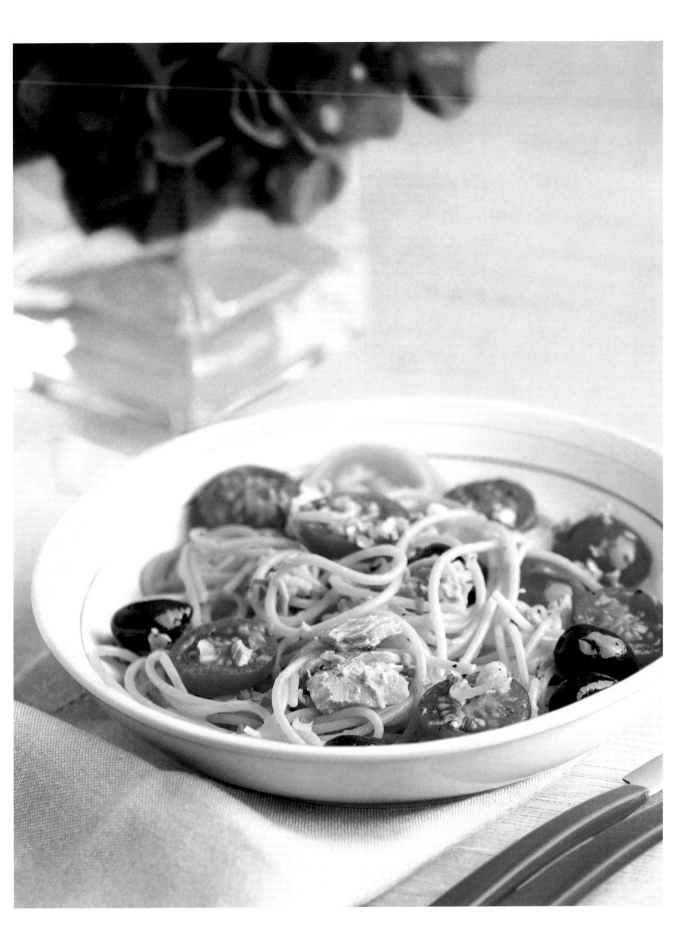

Chicken and Brie Ciabatta Pizza

Meal total
395
CALORIES

1 small ciabatta baguette
or 2 ciabatta rolls

30 ml (2 tbsp) sun-dried
tomato pesto

250 ml (1 cup) cooked chicken,
cut into strips

125 ml (½ cup) roasted peppers,
drained and sliced

60 ml (¼ cup) fresh basil,
chopped

100 g Brie, cut into slices

Pepper to taste

Prep time **20 minutes**

Cook time **8 minutes**

Serves **4**

PER SERVING	
Calories	395
Protein	23 g
Fat	15 g
Carbohydrates	42 g
Fibre	2 g
Iron	4 mg
Calcium	56 mg
Sodium	784 mg

1. Preheat the oven to 230°C
(450°F).

2. Cut the baguette in half and
slice each half lengthwise. Lightly
press down on the centre of each
half so that you can easily lay out
the toppings. Place the bread on a
baking sheet lined with parchment
paper.

3. Brush the bread with pesto.

4. Top the bread with chicken,
peppers, half of the basil and Brie.
Season with pepper.

5. Bake for 8 minutes, until the
cheese melts and the bread
is golden-brown.

6. Sprinkle each serving with
the rest of the basil.

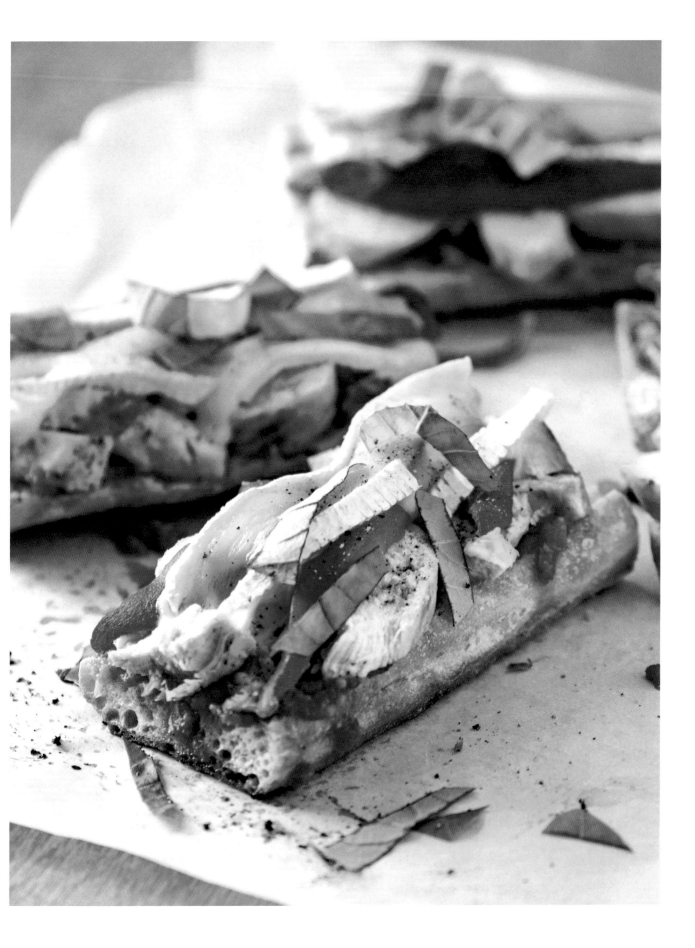

Deliciously Vegetarian

Eating vegetarian shouldn't prevent you from enjoying a variety of mouth-watering recipes. Out with the green salads sans vinaigrette, in with the lasagna primavera, souffléd pizzaiola omelette, tofu bourguignon and other meat-free delicacies.

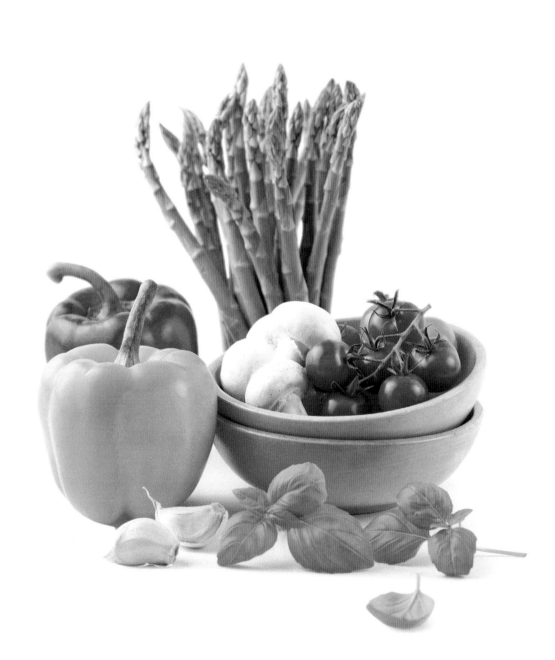

Lasagna Primavera

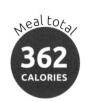

2 yellow zucchinis

2 green zucchinis

1 medium eggplant

2 red peppers

1 red onion

10 mushrooms

30 ml (2 tbsp) olive oil

Salt and pepper to taste

9 lasagna sheets

45 ml (3 tbsp) butter

45 ml (3 tbsp) flour

500 ml (2 cups) milk

500 ml (2 cups) light
mozzarella, shredded

1 can (680 ml) tomato
sauce

Prep time **20 minutes**

Cook time **40 minutes**

Serves **6 to 8**

PER SERVING	
Calories	362
Protein	17 g
Fat	15 g
Carbohydrates	42 g
Fibre	6 g
Iron	2 mg
Calcium	346 mg
Sodium	275 mg

1. Set the oven to broil.

2. Slice the vegetables and place them on a baking sheet lined with parchment paper. Drizzle with oil and season with salt and pepper. Bake for 2 to 3 minutes on each side. Remove from the oven and set aside. Set the oven to 180°C (350°F).

3. Cook the lasagna *al dente* in a pot of boiling, salted water. Drain.

4. In another pot, melt the butter over medium heat. Sprinkle with flour. Cook for 1 to 2 minutes, stirring with a wooden spoon, without letting the flour brown. Whisk in the milk and bring to a boil. Whisk constantly and cook until the mixture thickens.

5. Remove the pot from the heat and add 250 ml (1 cup) of cheese. Season with salt and pepper.

6. Spread half of the tomato sauce over the bottom of a 33 cm x 23 cm (13 in x 9 in) baking dish. Place three lasagna sheets across the sauce and half of the vegetable slices on the lasagna sheets. Repeat with three more lasagna sheets and the rest of the vegetables. Top with the rest of the tomato sauce. Cover with the last three lasagna sheets and top with the cheese sauce. Sprinkle with the remaining cheese. Bake for 30 to 40 minutes.

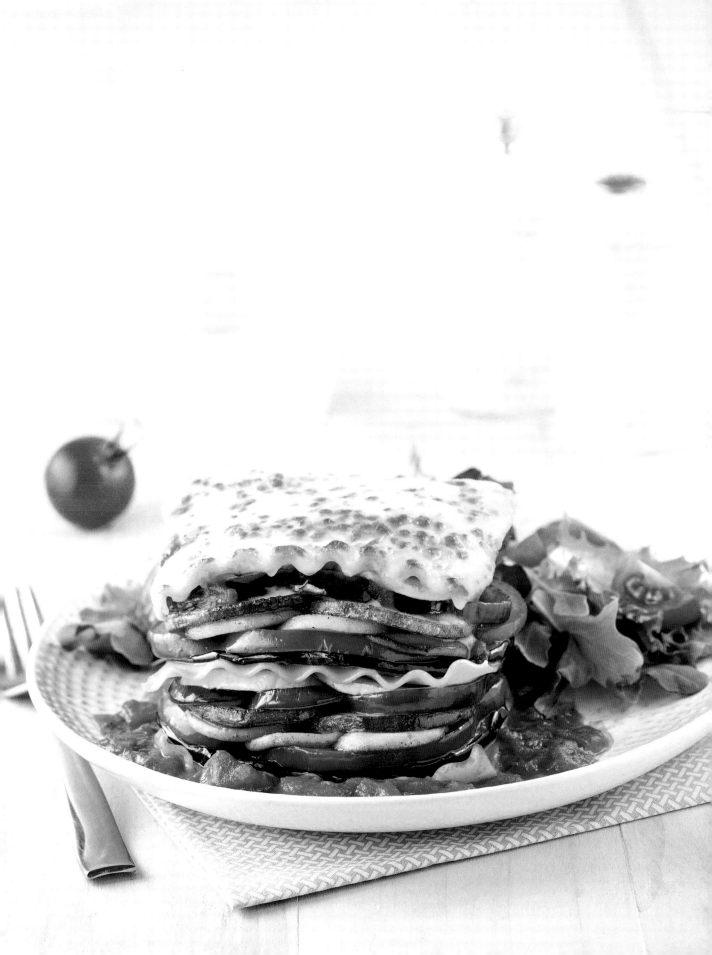

Tofu Pad Thai

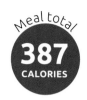

Meal total
387
CALORIES

For the pad Thai:

100 g wide rice noodles

45 ml (3 tbsp) sesame oil (untoasted)

3 eggs, beaten

250 g firm tofu, cut into cubes

1 onion, chopped

10 ml (2 tsp) garlic, minced

2 carrots, cut into thin julienne strips

250 ml (1 cup) bean sprouts

30 ml (2 tbsp) cilantro leaves

60 ml (¼ cup) roasted peanuts

For the sauce:

125 ml (½ cup) vegetable stock

45 ml (3 tbsp) soy sauce

30 ml (2 tbsp) lime juice

15 ml (1 tbsp) honey

Prep time **30 minutes**

Cook time **8 minutes**

Serves **4**

PER SERVING	
Calories	387
Protein	16 g
Fat	21 g
Carbohydrates	35 g
Fibre	2 g
Iron	2 mg
Calcium	76 mg
Sodium	1,015 mg

1. Prepare the noodles according to the instructions on the packaging, but make sure to leave them slightly crunchy. Drain.

2. Mix the sauce ingredients in a bowl.

3. Heat 15 ml (1 tbsp) of oil in a frying pan or wok over medium heat. Add the eggs and tilt the pan in all directions to fully cover the bottom, forming a thin omelette. Cook for 1 minute, until the sides begin to brown. Flip and cook the other side. Transfer to a plate. Roll up the omelette and cut it into thin rounds.

4. Heat the rest of the oil in the same pan over medium heat. Cook the tofu for 2 to 3 minutes, until it's golden-brown on all sides.

5. Add the onion, garlic and carrots. Cook for 2 minutes.

6. Add the sauce, bean sprouts and noodles. Cook for another 2 to 3 minutes.

7. Divide the pad Thai into bowls. Top each serving with omelette rolls, cilantro and peanuts.

Did you know?

The many benefits of tofu

Soy, the basic ingredient of tofu, is a high-quality source of protein. Of the legumes, soy contains the highest amount of complete protein— proteins containing all nine of the essential amino acids. This means that tofu can easily replace the meat in your meals once or twice a week. It is low in saturated fat and even has good fat that helps reduce blood cholesterol levels. Tofu also contains significant amounts of phytoestrogens, which are plant hormones that are thought to help reduce the severity of menopausal symptoms. Tofu can be eaten grilled, sautéed, fried or stewed. It can also be crumbled into soups and salads.

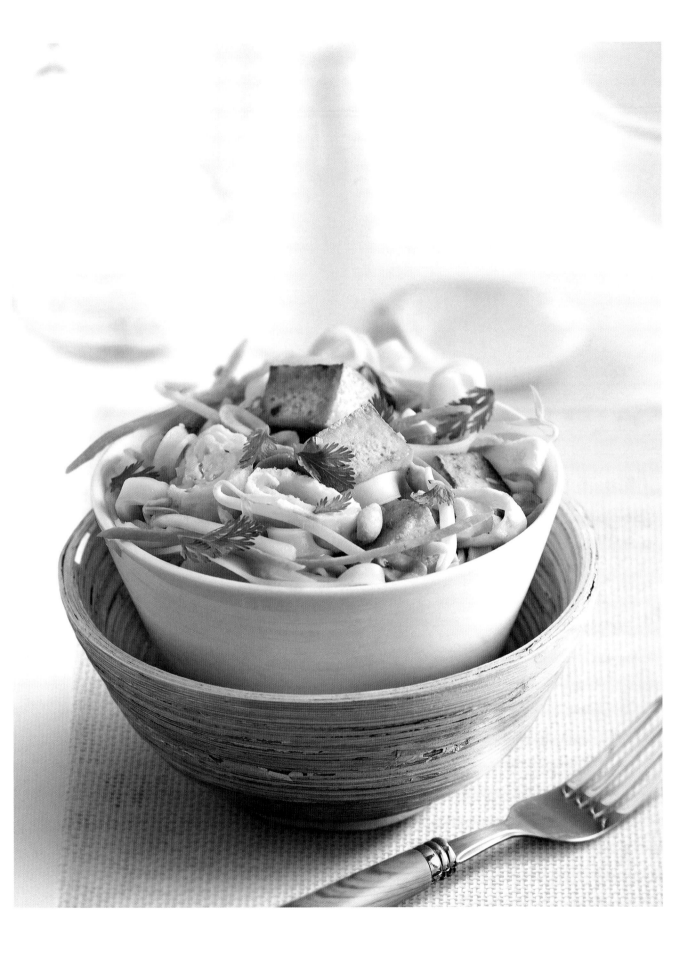

Souffléd Pizzaiola Omelette

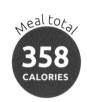

Meal total
358
CALORIES

For the omelette:

Olive oil

6 eggs, yolks and whites separated

10 ml (2 tsp) fresh chives, chopped

1.25 ml (¼ tsp) salt

Pepper to taste

3 drops of tabasco

For the vegetable toppings:

10 ml (2 tsp) olive oil

500 ml (2 cups) mushrooms, cut into wedges

1 garlic clove, minced

1 sprig thyme, chopped

½ pepper, cut into strips

250 ml (1 cup) strained tomatoes

Salt and pepper to taste

500 ml (2 cups) light mozzarella

Fresh basil to taste

Prep time **35 minutes**

Cook time **18 minutes**

Serves **4**

PER SERVING	
Calories	299
Protein	28 g
Fat	19 g
Carbohydrates	8 g
Fibre	1 g
Iron	1 mg
Calcium	488 mg
Sodium	821 mg

1. Preheat the oven to 205°C (400°F).

2. Use a brush to oil a non-stick ovenproof skillet, about 25 cm (10 in) in diameter.

3. Use an electric mixer to whip the egg whites until stiff peaks form. In another large bowl, beat the egg yolks. Gradually add the egg whites to the yolks, mixing gently. Add the rest of the omelette ingredients.

4. Pour the mixture into the skillet and bake for 8 minutes, until the eggs begin to set.

5. While the eggs are cooking, heat the oil in another frying pan over high heat. Sauté the mushrooms, garlic and thyme for 4 minutes, until the mushrooms are golden-brown. Add the pepper and cook for a few more seconds. Add the strained tomatoes, salt and pepper.

6. Remove the omelette from the oven and gently distribute the toppings over the surface. Sprinkle with cheese. Put back in the oven and bake for another 10 minutes, until the cheese has melted and the omelette is fully set.

7. Sprinkle each serving with basil.

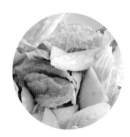

Try it with...

Green Salad With Lemon Vinaigrette
Per serving: 59 calories
In a salad bowl, mix 15 ml (1 tbsp) olive oil with 15 ml (1 tbsp) lemon juice. Add 1 head romaine lettuce, shredded, and 1 green apple, cut into thin slices. Toss well and sprinkle with fleur de sel.

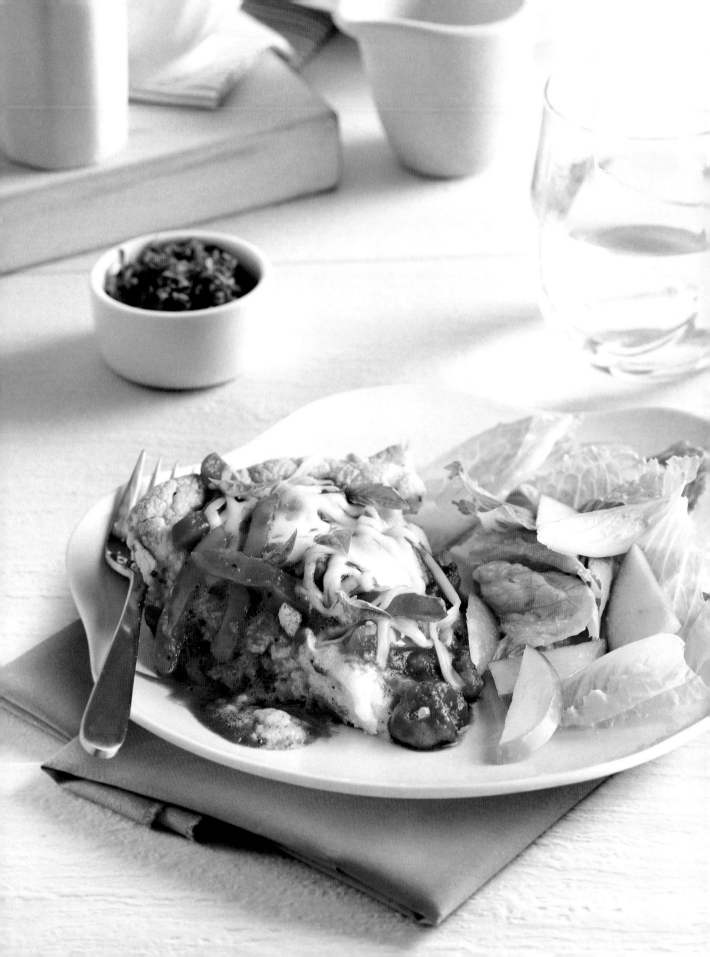

Cheesy Red Bean Spaghetti Squash

Meal total
395
CALORIES

2 small spaghetti squash

15 ml (1 tbsp) olive oil

Salt and pepper to taste

1 onion, chopped

2 tomatoes, diced

1 can (540 ml) red beans, rinsed and drained

3 pepper halves, various colours, diced

310 ml (1 ¼ cups) tomato sauce with herbs

30 ml (2 tbsp) fresh basil, chopped

15 ml (1 tbsp) fresh thyme, chopped

250 ml (1 cup) light mozzarella, shredded

Prep time **20 minutes**

Cook time **55 minutes**

Serves **4**

PER SERVING	
Calories	395
Protein	20 g
Fat	11 g
Carbohydrates	59 g
Fibre	12 g
Iron	5 mg
Calcium	361 mg
Sodium	550 mg

1. Preheat the oven to 190°C (375°F).

2. Cut the spaghetti squash in half lengthwise. Remove the seeds and strands.

3. Place the squash on a baking sheet, flesh side up. Drizzle with half of the olive oil. Season with salt and pepper.

4. Bake for 40 to 45 minutes, until the flesh of the squash shreds easily with a fork.

5. Heat the rest of the oil in a frying pan over medium heat. Cook the onion for 1 minute.

6. Add the tomatoes, red beans, peppers, tomato sauce and herbs. Bring to a boil. Season with salt and pepper.

7. Pour the red bean mixture into the squash halves. Cover with cheese. Bake for 15 minutes.

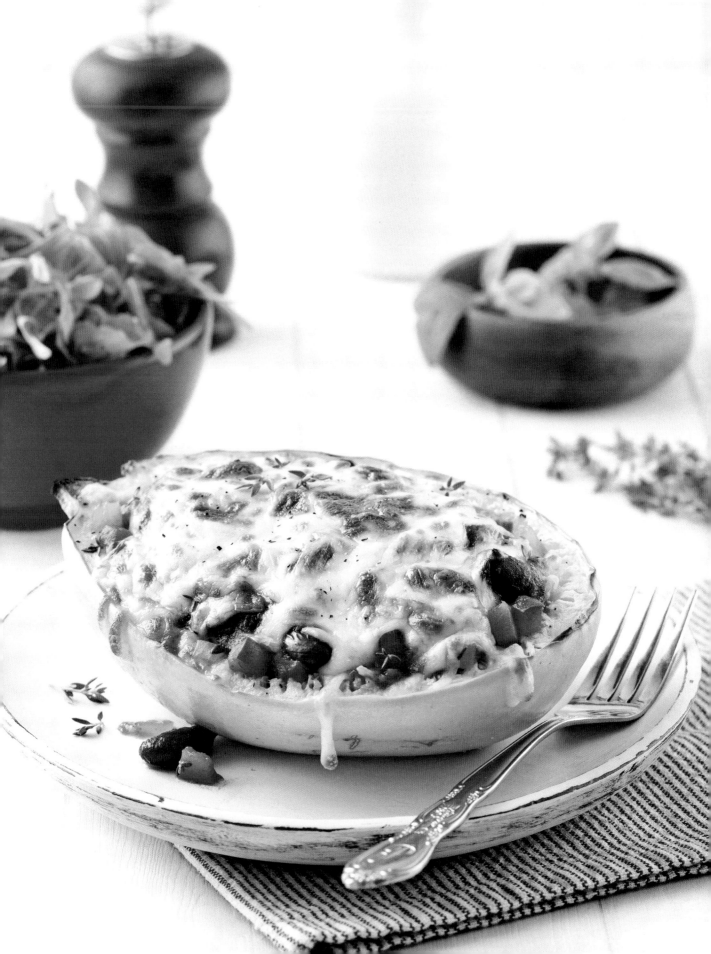

Vegetarian Meat Loaf

Meal total
321
CALORIES

180 ml (¾ cup) ketchup

30 ml (2 tbsp) brown sugar

1 can (540 ml) white beans, rinsed and drained

1 block (300 g) soft silken tofu

60 ml (¼ cup) tomato paste

15 ml (1 tbsp) paprika

3 eggs

250 ml (1 cup) quick-cooking oats

1 carrot, grated

45 ml (3 tbsp) fresh parsley, chopped

15 ml (1 tbsp) fresh thyme, chopped

15 ml (1 tbsp) salad seasoning

125 ml (½ cup) Parmesan, grated

Pepper to taste

Prep time **20 minutes**

Cook time **50 minutes**

Serves **6**

PER SERVING	
Calories	321
Protein	18 g
Fat	8 g
Carbohydrates	47 g
Fibre	8 g
Iron	5 mg
Calcium	193 mg
Sodium	848 mg

1. Preheat the oven to 190°C (375°F).

2. In a bowl, mix the ketchup with the brown sugar.

3. In a food processor, puree the beans with the tofu, tomato paste, paprika and eggs.

4. Transfer the bean mixture to a bowl. Add the oats, carrot, herbs, salad seasoning and Parmesan. Season with pepper and stir.

5. Pour the mixture into a loaf pan lined with parchment paper. Smooth out the surface with the back of a spoon. Top with the ketchup mixture.

6. Bake for 50 minutes to 1 hour.

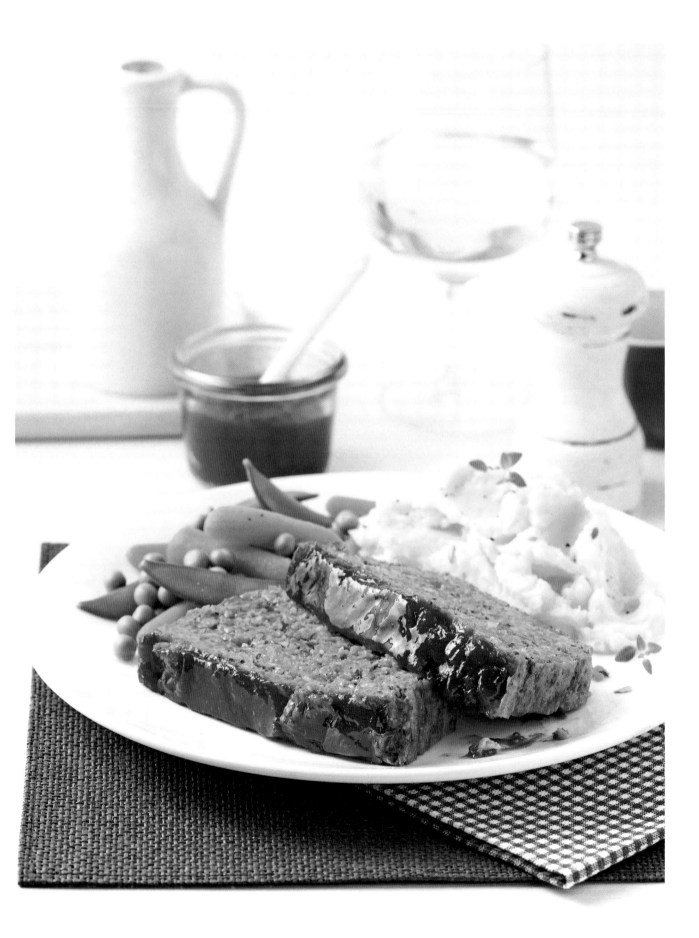

Tofu Bourguignon

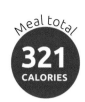

Meal total
321
CALORIES

30 ml (2 tbsp) olive oil

1 block (454 g) firm tofu, cut into large cubes

250 ml (1 cup) pearl onions, peeled

250 ml (1 cup) carrots, sliced

500 ml (2 cups) cremini mushrooms, cut into wedges

30 ml (2 tbsp) tomato paste

125 ml (½ cup) red wine

750 ml (3 cups) vegetable stock

1 garlic clove, minced

Salt and pepper to taste

1 sprig thyme

30 ml (2 tbsp) cornstarch

30 ml (2 tbsp) water

Prep time **30 minutes**

Cook time **30 minutes**

Serves **4**

PER SERVING	
Calories	321
Protein	22 g
Fat	16 g
Carbohydrates	17 g
Fibre	3 g
Iron	4 mg
Calcium	138 mg
Sodium	523 mg

1. Heat 15 ml (1 tbsp) of oil in a non-stick frying pan over high heat. Brown the tofu cubes on each side. Place on a paper towel and set aside.

2. Add the rest of the oil to a pot and cook the onions over medium heat for 2 to 3 minutes. Add the carrots and cook until tender.

3. Add the mushrooms, tomato paste, red wine, stock, garlic and tofu. Season with salt and pepper, and add the sprig of thyme. Bring to a boil, and then cover and let simmer over low heat for 30 minutes, until the vegetables are tender.

4. In a small bowl, dissolve the cornstarch in the water. Add to the pot and mix. Bring to a boil and gently stir until the bourguignon thickens.

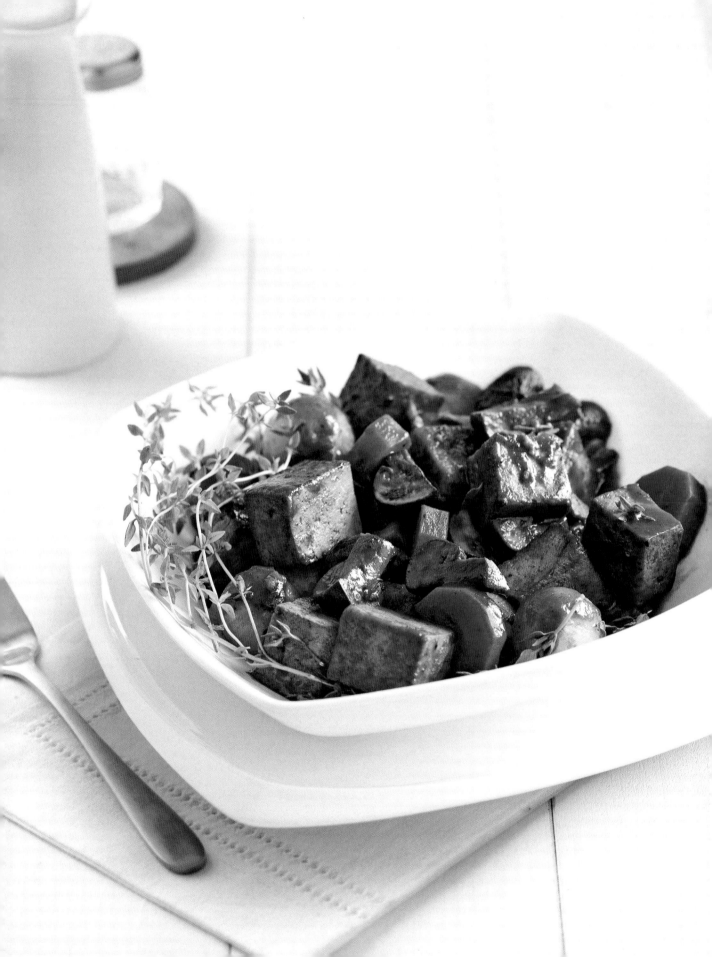

Orange, Cashew and Tofu Stir-Fry

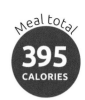

Meal total
395 CALORIES

1 block (454 g) firm tofu

1 carrot

15 ml (1 tbsp) canola oil

10 ml (2 tsp) garlic, minced

1 can (227 ml) water chestnuts, drained

8 shiitake mushrooms, sliced

125 ml (½ cup) cashews

A few leaves cilantro (optional)

For the orange sauce:

250 ml (1 cup) orange juice

45 ml (3 tbsp) soy sauce

15 ml (1 tbsp) cornstarch

Salt and pepper to taste

Prep time **25 minutes**

Cook time **8 minutes**

Serves **4**

PER SERVING	
Calories	395
Protein	25 g
Fat	21 g
Carbohydrates	29 g
Fibre	4 g
Iron	5 mg
Calcium	127 mg
Sodium	788 mg

1. Cut the tofu into roughly 1.5 cm (⅔ in) cubes and the carrot into thin julienne strips.

2. Heat the oil in a frying pan or wok over medium heat. Brown the tofu cubes for 2 to 3 minutes. Remove from the pan.

3. In the same pan, cook the garlic, water chestnuts, shiitake mushrooms, carrot and cashews for 3 to 4 minutes.

4. In a bowl, mix the orange juice with the soy sauce and cornstarch. Season with salt and pepper. Pour into the pan and stir until it begins to boil.

5. Add the tofu and heat for 1 more minute.

6. Sprinkle each serving with cilantro if desired.

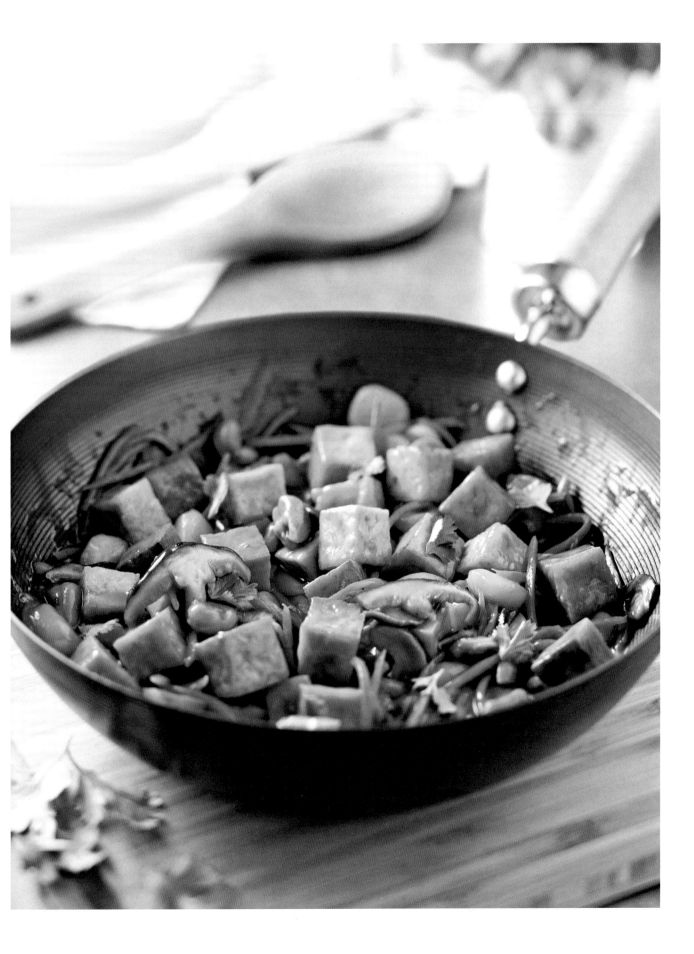

Not-So-Guilty Desserts

Maintaining or achieving a healthy weight doesn't always mean saying no to sugar! In this section, you'll discover a selection of light yet decadent desserts that you can savour without the regret.

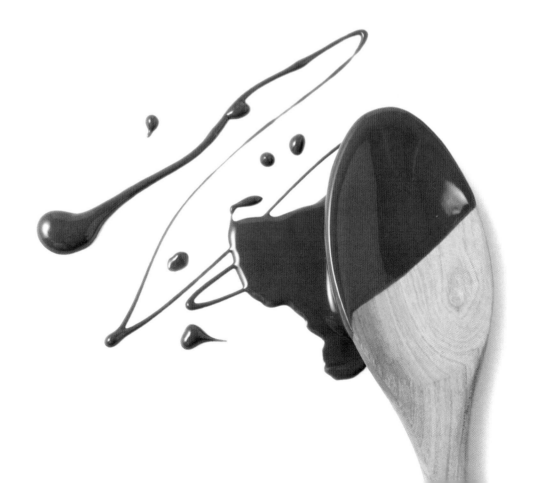

Maple Banana Bread

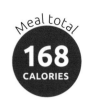

250 ml (1 cup) all-purpose flour

125 ml (½ cup) whole wheat flour

80 ml (⅓ cup) ground flaxseed

15 ml (1 tbsp) baking powder

2.5 ml (½ tsp) baking soda

1.25 ml (¼ tsp) salt

2 eggs

125 ml (½ cup) maple syrup

5 ml (1 tsp) vanilla extract

30 ml (2 tbsp) canola oil

375 ml (1 ½ cups) bananas, pureed (about 2 bananas)

15 ml (1 tbsp) whole flaxseed

60 ml (¼ cup) walnuts, chopped

60 ml (¼ cup) dark chocolate (70%), chopped (optional)

Prep time **20 minutes**

Cook time **50 minutes**

Serves **16**

PER SERVING	
Calories	168
Protein	4 g
Fat	7 g
Carbohydrates	24 g
Fibre	2 g
Iron	1 mg
Calcium	30 mg
Sodium	135 mg

1. Preheat the oven to 180°C (350°F).

2. In a bowl, mix both flours with the ground flaxseed, baking powder, baking soda and salt.

3. In another bowl, beat the eggs with the maple syrup, vanilla, oil and pureed bananas. Gradually add the dry ingredients and stir until evenly mixed.

4. Line a 20 cm x 10 cm (8 in x 4 in) loaf pan with parchment paper and pour in the batter. Smooth out the surface.

5. Top the batter with whole flaxseed and walnuts. Bake for 50 minutes to 1 hour, until a toothpick inserted into the centre comes out clean. Remove the pan from the oven and let cool on a rack.

6. Top the banana bread with the chocolate if desired.

7. Cut the bread into eight slices and cut each slice in half.

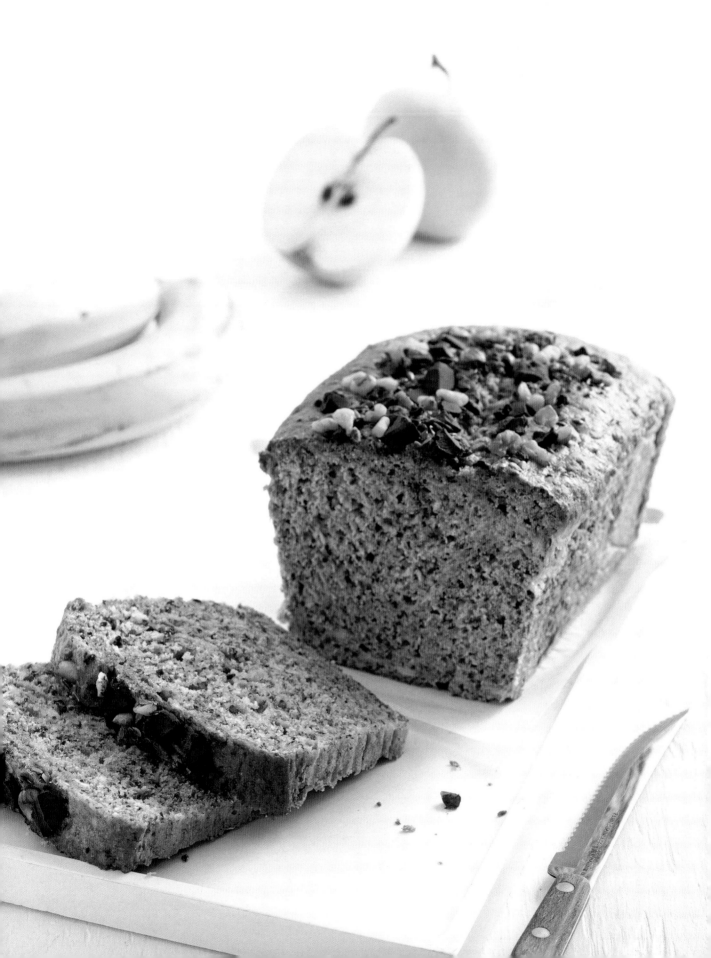

Chocolate, Banana and Pear Crumble Cups

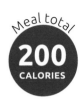

Meal total
200
CALORIES

6 chocolate tea biscuits

30 ml (2 tbsp) butter

2 bananas

1 pear

15 ml (1 tbsp) lemon juice

60 ml (¼ cup) 2% milk

1 bar (100 g) milk chocolate

Prep time **15 minutes**

Cook time **5 minutes**

Serves **6**

PER SERVING	
Calories	200
Protein	2 g
Fat	9 g
Carbohydrates	28 g
Fibre	2 g
Iron	0 mg
Calcium	42 mg
Sodium	50 mg

1. Preheat the oven to 180°C (350°F).

2. Crush the chocolate biscuits in a bowl and mix with the butter. Distribute the mixture onto a baking sheet lined with parchment paper. Bake for 5 to 6 minutes.

3. Dice the bananas and pear. Place in another bowl and gently mix with the lemon juice. Divide into six dessert cups.

4. Pour the milk into a pot and bring to a boil. Remove from heat.

5. Add the chocolate to the hot milk. Stir until the chocolate is melted.

6. Divide the chocolate into the cups and garnish each serving with the crumble.

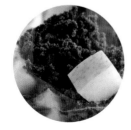

Try it with...

Homemade crumble

How about making your own classic crumble for these dessert cups? This basic recipe is a cinch. You'll need equal parts flour, brown sugar and butter. Thoroughly mix the dry ingredients and then gradually add the melted butter. Work with a fork or your fingers until the dough is grainy. For chocolate crumble, add 45 ml (3 tbsp) of cacao powder to the dry ingredients. Homemade crumble needs to bake at 180°C (350°F) for 20 to 25 minutes to be properly crispy.

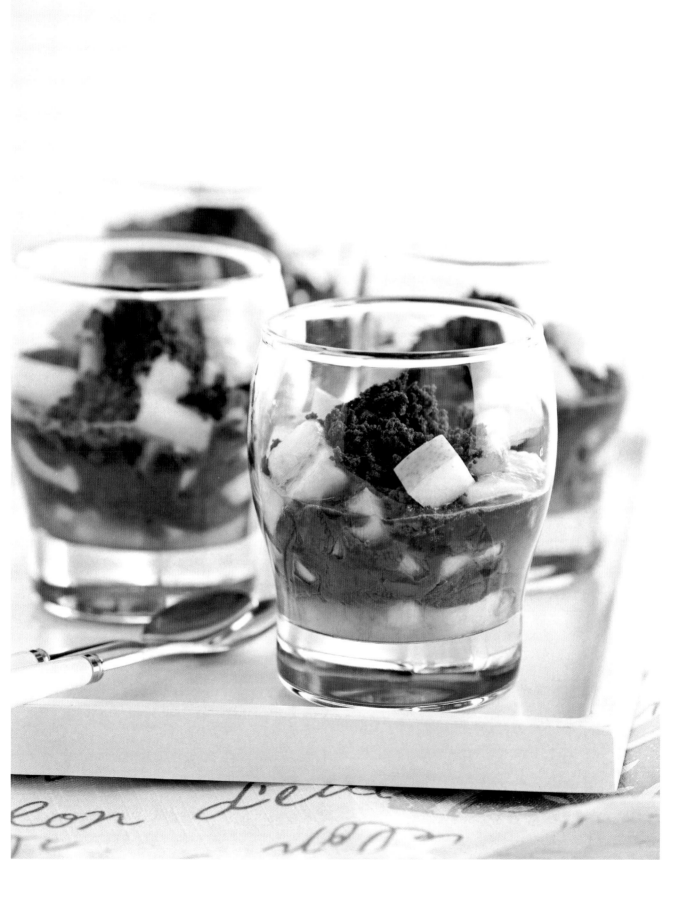

Pineapple Walnut Carrot Cake

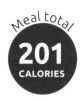

Meal total
201
CALORIES

For the cake:

500 ml (2 cups) whole wheat flour

125 ml (½ cup) brown sugar

30 ml (2 tbsp) baking powder

30 ml (2 tbsp) cinnamon

15 ml (1 tbsp) baking soda

10 ml (2 tsp) nutmeg

5 ml (1 tsp) ground ginger

1 pinch salt

3 eggs

250 ml (1 cup) unsweetened apple sauce

560 ml (2 ¼ cups) carrots, grated

125 ml (½ cup) diced pineapples, drained

60 ml (¼ cup) walnuts, chopped

For the whipped cream:

125 ml (½ cup) 35% whipping cream

15 ml (1 tbsp) powdered sugar

15 ml (1 tbsp) lemon zest

2 drops vanilla extract

Prep time **25 minutes**

Cook time **50 minutes**

Serves **12**

PER SERVING	
Calories	201
Protein	5 g
Fat	7 g
Carbohydrates	29 g
Fibre	4 g
Iron	1 mg
Calcium	49 mg
Sodium	474 mg

1. Preheat the oven to 180°C (350°F).

2. Mix the dry ingredients in a bowl. In another bowl, beat the eggs and add the apple sauce, carrots, pineapples and walnuts. Gradually add the dry ingredients and stir until evenly mixed.

3. Grease a 20 cm (8 in) square baking dish and pour in the batter. Bake for 50 minutes and then let cool.

4. While the cake is cooking, use an electric mixer to whip the cream at high speed. Add the powdered sugar, zest and vanilla.

5. Cut the cake into 12 squares and top each portion with a dollop of whipped cream.

Did you know?

You can replace fat with apple sauce

Strange as it may seem, apple sauce is a great substitute for fat. If your recipe calls for 250 ml (1 cup) of butter, margarine or oil, you can replace it with the same quantity of unsweetened apple sauce. You'll spare yourself the calories and fat, but your desserts will be just as delicious and tender!

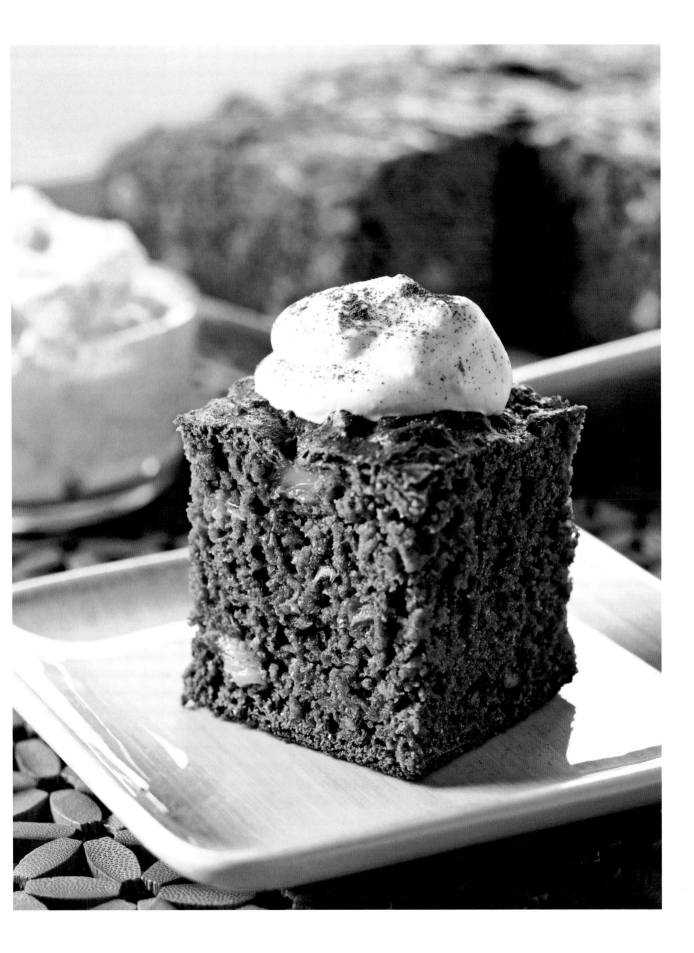

Mini Chocolate Lava Cakes

Meal total
140
CALORIES

135 g dark chocolate (70%), cut into pieces

80 ml (⅓ cup) unsalted butter

45 ml (3 tbsp) 2 % milk

60 ml (¼ cup) brown sugar

2 eggs

15 ml (1 tbsp) unbleached all-purpose flour

15 ml (1 tbsp) cornstarch

Prep time **15 minutes**

Refrigeration **1 hour**

Cook time **4 minutes**

Yields **12 mini cakes**

PER SERVING	
Calories	140
Protein	2 g
Fat	11 g
Carbohydrates	10 g
Fibre	1 g
Iron	1 mg
Calcium	19 mg
Sodium	21 mg

1. Place the chocolate and butter in a bowl. Microwave for 90 seconds. Add the milk and stir until evenly mixed. The heat from the butter will continue to melt the chocolate. Set aside.

2. In a bowl, whisk together the brown sugar and eggs for 2 minutes until light in colour and fluffy. Add the flour and cornstarch. Continue to whisk until smooth.

3. Add the prepared chocolate to the egg mixture and stir with a rubber spatula until smooth. Refrigerate the batter for at least 1 hour.

4. When ready to cook, preheat the oven to 205°C (400°F).

5. Use butter or vegetable oil spray to grease the cups of a muffin tin. Place about 15 ml (1 tbsp) of batter into each cup. Bake for 4 to 5 minutes. The centre should remain melted. Gently remove from the muffin tin and serve immediately.

Did you know?

Pleasure and health can go hand in hand!
Healthy eating can definitely include partaking in your fair share of desserts, chocolate and calories. Portion size and frequency are obviously very important concepts to keep in mind, which is why we are offering you this recipe for mini indulgence!

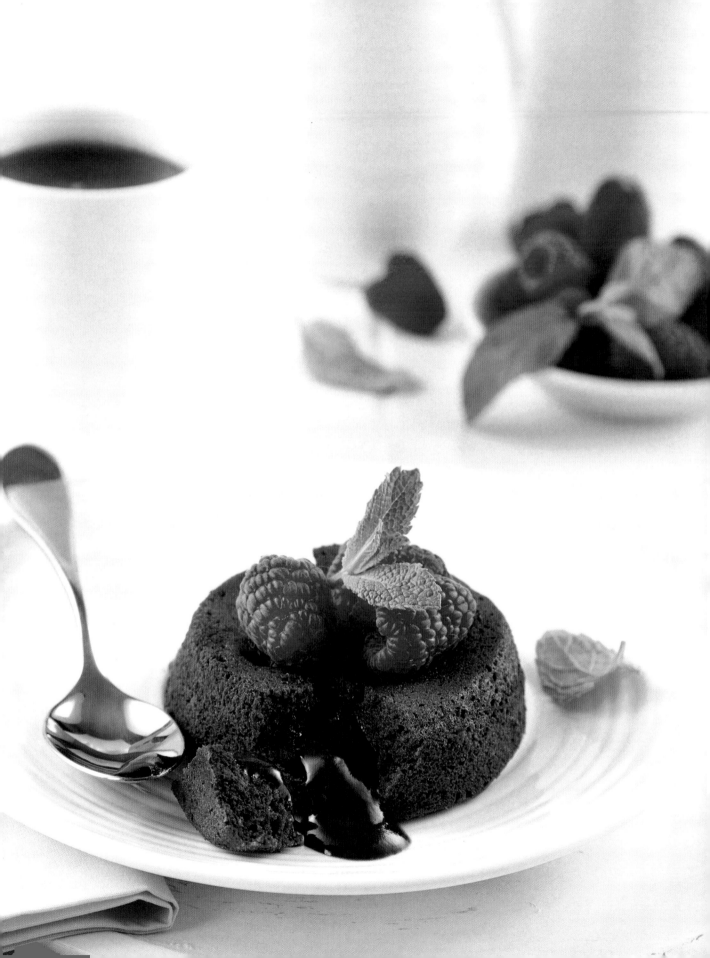

Mini Chai Lime Cupcakes

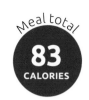

Meal total
83
CALORIES

80 ml (⅓ cup) butter

2 chai tea bags

160 ml (⅔ cup) flour

5 ml (1 tsp) baking powder

15 ml (1 tbsp) lime zest

1 pinch salt

3 eggs

125 ml (½ cup) sugar

2 to 3 drops vanilla extract

Prep time **15 minutes**

Cook time **10 minutes**

Yields **24 mini cupcakes**

PER SERVING	
Calories	62
Protein	1 g
Fat	3 g
Carbohydrates	7 g
Fibre	0 g
Iron	0 mg
Calcium	14 mg
Sodium	14 mg

1. Preheat the oven to 180°C (350°F).

2. Melt the butter in a small pot or in the microwave. Cut open the tea bags and pour the contents into the melted butter. Cover with plastic wrap and let infuse for 10 minutes. Use a fine strainer to filter the butter.

3. In a bowl, mix the flour with the baking powder, lime zest and salt.

4. Use an electric mixer to beat the eggs with the sugar and vanilla until light in colour. Gently add the dry ingredients and the butter.

5. Grease the cups of a muffin tin, or line them with paper baking cups. Divide the batter into the cups. Bake for 10 to 12 minutes.

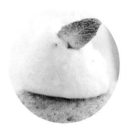

Try it with...

Lime-Flavoured Whipped Cream
Per serving: 21 calories
Whip 125 ml (½ cup) 35% whipping cream, 30 ml (2 tbsp) sugar and 5 ml (1 tsp) lime zest until stiff peaks form. Top the cupcakes.

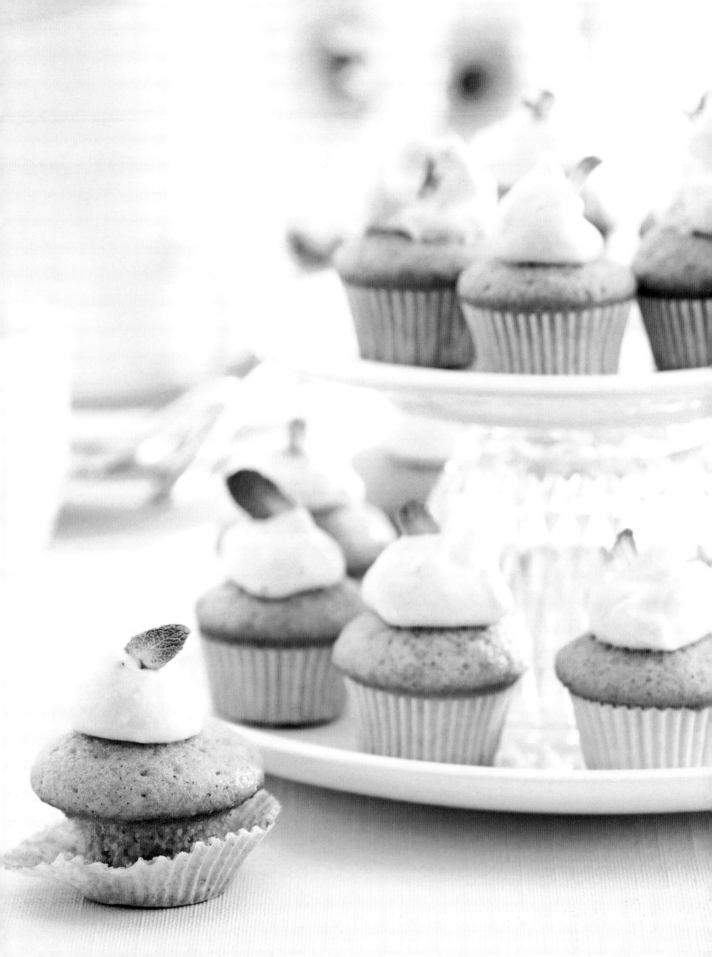

Chocolate Strawberry Yogourt Squares

Meal total
199
CALORIES

180 ml (¾ cup) brown sugar

375 ml (1 ½ cups) all-purpose flour

45 ml (3 tbsp) cacao powder

1 to 2 pinches cinnamon

60 ml (¼ cup) walnuts, chopped

250 ml (1 cup) oats

60 g dark chocolate (70%)

90 ml (about ⅓ cup) canola oil

125 ml (½ cup) orange juice

1 ½ packets (7 g each) unflavoured gelatin

500 ml (2 cups) strawberry yogourt (0%)

Prep time **20 minutes**

Cook time **10 minutes**

Refrigeration **2 hours**

Serves **16**

PER SERVING	
Calories	199
Protein	6 g
Fat	8 g
Carbohydrates	27 g
Fibre	2 g
Iron	1 mg
Calcium	43 mg
Sodium	16 mg

1. Preheat the oven to 180°C (350°F).

2. In a bowl, mix the brown sugar with the flour, cacao powder, cinnamon, walnuts and oats.

3. Melt the chocolate in a pot or in the microwave. Add the oil. Add the melted chocolate to the dry ingredients and mix thoroughly.

4. Grease a 20 cm (8 in) square baking dish and pour in the mixture. Press to even out the surface of the crust. Bake for 10 to 12 minutes. Remove the dish from the oven and let cool completely.

5. Pour the orange juice into a bowl. Add the gelatin and let bloom for 3 minutes. Microwave for a few seconds.

6. Place the yogourt in another bowl. Gradually whisk in the orange juice. Pour the mixture into the baking dish, on top of the crust. Cover and refrigerate for 2 hours. Cut into 16 squares.

Also try it...

As a nut-free recipe
Do you steer clear of nuts because of an allergy? Don't write off this recipe just yet! Simply replace the walnuts with the same quantity of oats—the result will be just as delicious.

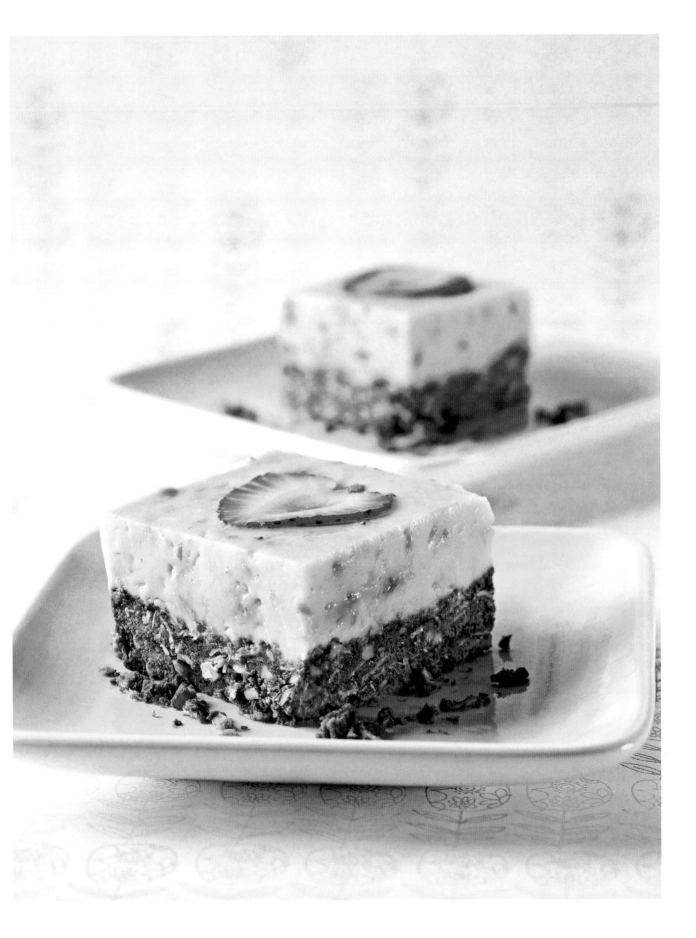

Lemon Tiramisu

Meal total
196
CALORIES

2 egg yolks

60 ml (¼ cup) sugar

125 ml (½ cup) mascarpone

180 ml (¾ cup) quark
or ricotta cheese

90 ml (6 tbsp) lemon juice

2 lemons (zest)

250 ml (1 cup) 35%
whipping cream

10 ladyfinger cookies,
cut in half

Prep time **20 minutes**

Refrigeration **8 hours**

Serves **10**

PER SERVING	
Calories	196
Protein	5 g
Fat	14 g
Carbohydrates	13 g
Fibre	0 g
Iron	0 mg
Calcium	69 mg
Sodium	41 mg

1. Use an electric mixer to beat the egg yolks with 30 ml (2 tbsp) of sugar until light in colour and fluffy.

2. Add the mascarpone and mix well. Add the quark or ricotta cheese and mix until smooth. Add 30 ml (2 tbsp) of lemon juice and the lemon zest. Mix and set aside.

3. Use an electric mixer to whip the cream until soft peaks form. Add the rest of the sugar and continue to whip until stiff peaks form.

4. Gently fold the whipped cream into the cheese mixture with a rubber spatula until evenly mixed.

5. Pour the rest of the lemon juice into a large deep plate. Quickly dip the cookies one at a time into the juice so that they become lightly saturated. Distribute the cookie halves into the bottom of ten dessert cups. Cover the cookies with the cheese mixture and even out the surface with a rubber spatula.

6. Refrigerate for at least 8 hours before serving.

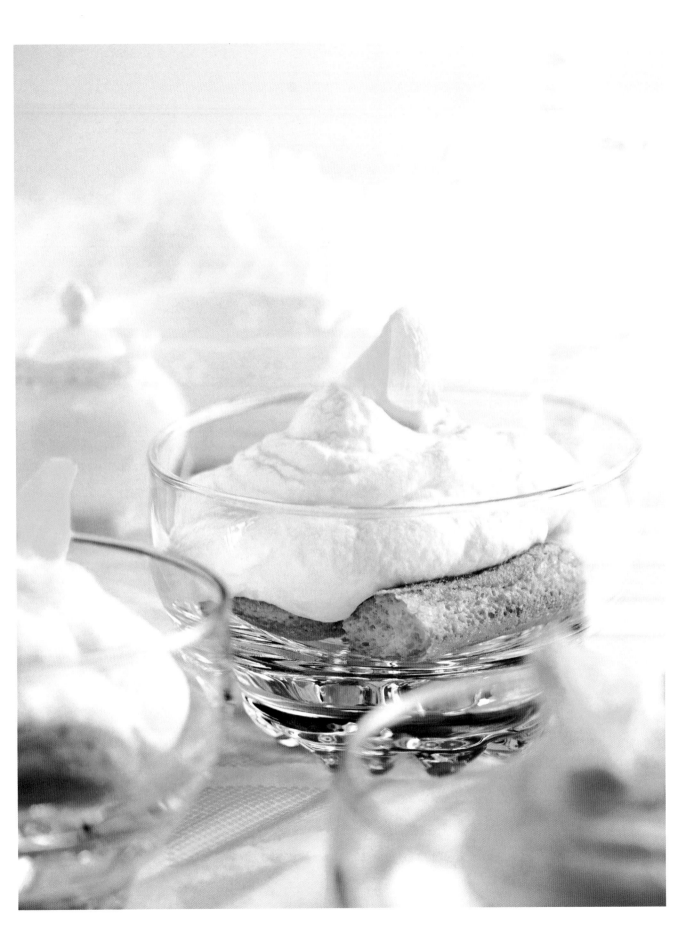

Blueberry and Orange Muffins

Meal total
173
CALORIES

250 ml (1 cup) unbleached all-purpose flour

250 ml (1 cup) whole wheat flour

20 ml (4 tsp) baking powder

60 ml (¼ cup) butter or non-hydrogenated margarine

125 ml (½ cup) brown sugar

2 eggs

250 ml (1 cup) 2 % milk

375 ml (1 ½ cups) blueberries, fresh or frozen

30 ml (2 tbsp) orange zest

Prep time **20 minutes**

Cook time **15 minutes**

Yields **10 to 12 muffins**

PER SERVING	
Calories	173
Protein	5 g
Fat	6 g
Carbohydrates	26 g
Fibre	2 g
Iron	1 mg
Calcium	44 mg
Sodium	157 mg

1. Preheat the oven to 205°C (400°F).

2. Oil the cups of a muffin tin, or line them with paper baking cups.

3. In a bowl, mix the flours with the baking powder.

4. In another bowl, use an electric mixer to beat the butter with the brown sugar until light in colour. Add the eggs and beat until evenly mixed. Add the milk.

5. Add the dry ingredients. Stir with a wooden spoon until evenly mixed, but avoid overmixing.

6. Add the blueberries and orange zest. Gently stir for a few seconds.

7. Pour the batter into the cups. Bake for 20 minutes, until a toothpick inserted into the centre of a muffin comes out clean.

8. Remove the muffin tin from the oven. Remove the muffins from the tin and let cool on a rack.

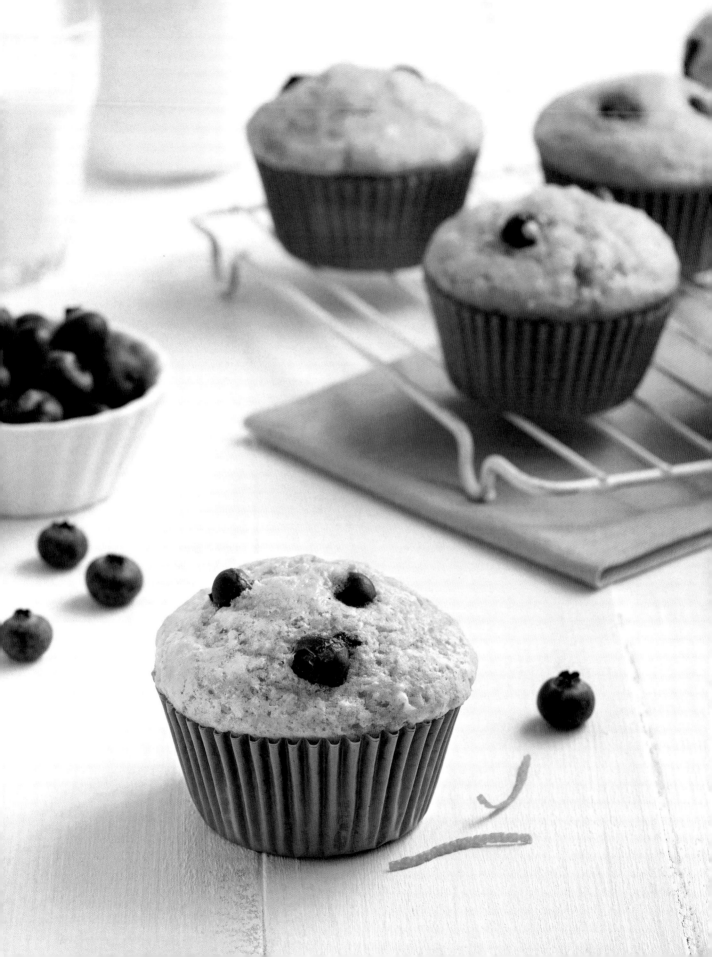

Lemon Meringue Pie

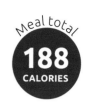

For the crust:

250 ml (1 cup) Graham cracker crumbs

30 ml (2 tbsp) sugar

45 ml (3 tbsp) melted butter

For the lemon topping:

330 ml (1 ⅓ cups) water

15 ml (1 tbsp) lemon zest

125 ml (½ cup) sugar

60 ml (¼ cup) cornstarch

2 egg yolks

45 ml (3 tbsp) lemon juice

For the Italian meringue:

125 ml (½ cup) sugar

30 ml (2 tbsp) water

2 egg whites

Prep time **45 minutes**

Cook time **8 minutes**

Serves **10**

PER SERVING	
Calories	188
Protein	2 g
Fat	5 g
Carbohydrates	34 g
Fibre	0 g
Iron	1 mg
Calcium	14 mg
Sodium	55 mg

1. Preheat the oven to 190°C (375°F).

2. In a bowl, mix the crust ingredients. Pour into a 20 cm (8 in) pie pan and press to even out the surface. Brown in the oven for 8 minutes. Let cool.

3. Place the water, zest and sugar in a pot and bring to a boil. Remove from heat.

4. In another bowl, whisk together the cornstarch, egg yolks and lemon juice. Strain.

5. Pour the sugar water onto the egg yolk mixture and whisk. Put back into the pot and let thicken over medium-high heat for 2 minutes, whisking constantly. Pour over the crust.

6. For the meringue, mix the sugar and water in a pot. Heat over high heat until the temperature reaches 116°C (240°F) on a cooking thermometer. Remove from heat.

7. Use an electric mixer to beat the egg whites until soft peaks form. Drizzle the syrup into the egg whites and continue to beat until stiff peaks form.

8. Distribute over the lemon topping. Brown under the broiler for 2 minutes.

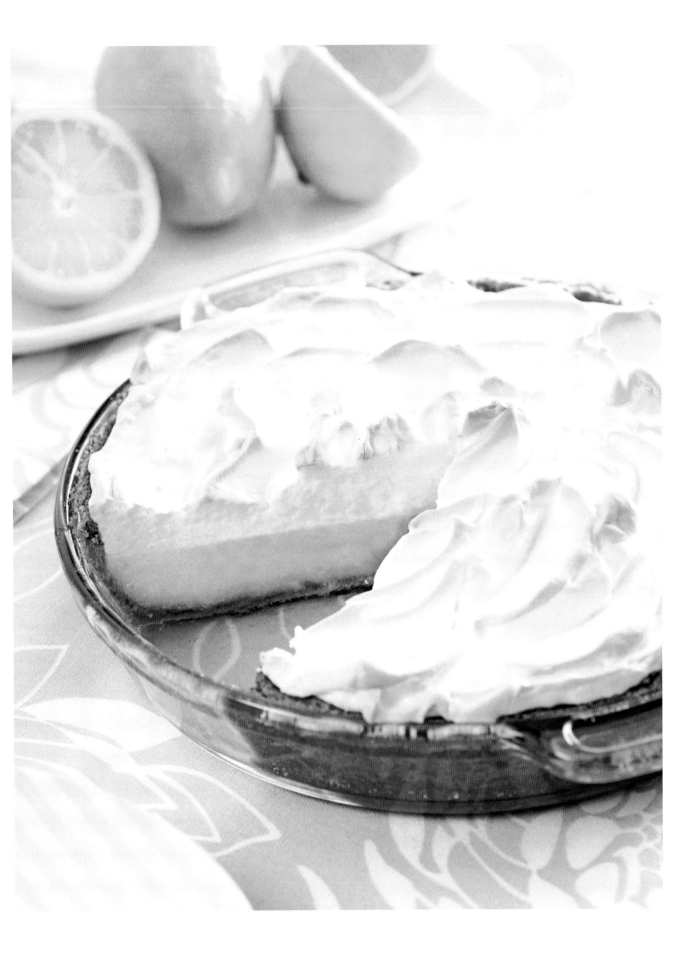

Molasses Cookies

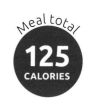

750 ml (3 cups) unbleached all-purpose flour

15 ml (1 tbsp) baking powder

5 ml (1 tsp) baking soda

5 ml (1 tsp) cinnamon

5 ml (1 tsp) ground ginger

125 ml (½ cup) butter or non-hydrogenated margarine

45 ml (3 tbsp) apple sauce

125 ml (½ cup) brown sugar

180 ml (¾ cup) molasses

1 egg

180 ml (¾ cup) 2 % milk

Prep time **20 minutes**

Cook time **10 minutes for each sheet**

Yields **30 cookies**

PER SERVING	
Calories	125
Protein	2 g
Fat	4 g
Carbohydrates	20 g
Fibre	0 g
Iron	1 mg
Calcium	32 mg
Sodium	103 mg

1. Preheat the oven to 180°C (350°F).

2. In a bowl, mix the flour with the baking powder, baking soda and spices.

3. In another bowl, use an electric mixer to combine the butter with the apple sauce, brown sugar and molasses until smooth. Add the egg and mix for a few seconds.

4. Alternate adding the dry ingredients and milk. Mix until smooth.

5. Line three baking sheets with parchment paper and form cookies using 30 ml (2 tbsp) of batter for each. Leave about 5 cm (2 in) of space between them.

6. Bake each baking sheet for 10 to 12 minutes. Do not overcook—the cookies are ready when they begin to set. Remove from the oven. Let the cookies cool on the baking sheets—they will finish cooking outside of the oven.

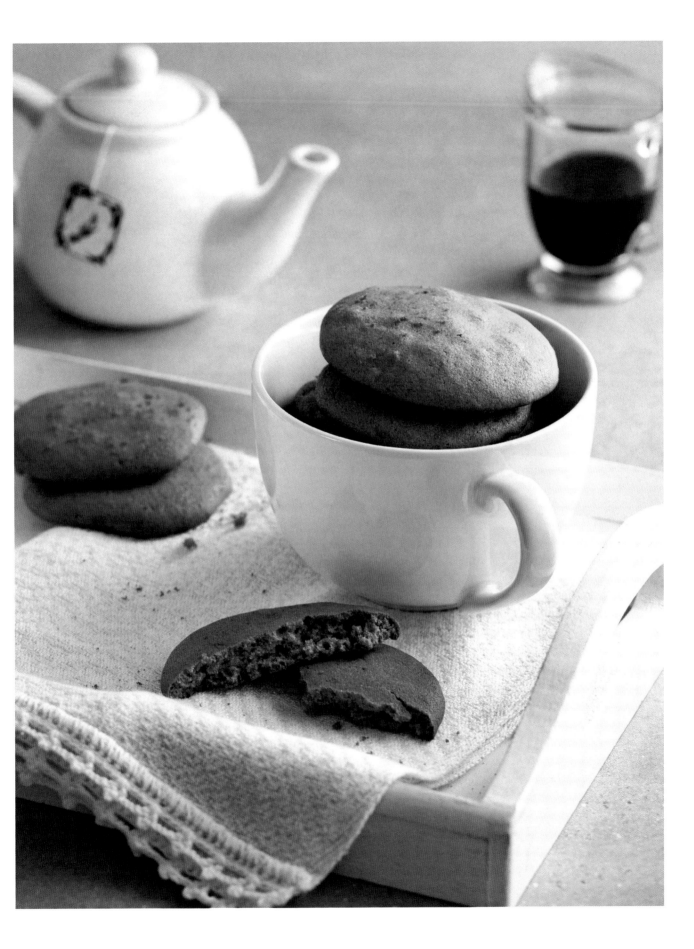

Chocolate and Cranberry Clusters

Meal total
101
CALORIES

200 g semi-sweet chocolate, cut into pieces

250 ml (1 cup) Rice Krispies

125 ml (½ cup) dried cranberries

1.25 ml (¼ tsp) cinnamon

1 pinch ground cardamom

Prep time **15 minutes**

Refrigeration **1 hour**

Yields **12 clusters**

PER SERVING	
Calories	101
Protein	1 g
Fat	5 g
Carbohydrates	16 g
Fibre	1 g
Iron	1 mg
Calcium	7 mg
Sodium	2 mg

1. Melt the chocolate in a bain-marie water bath. Remove from heat.

2. Add the rest of the ingredients and stir.

3. On a baking sheet lined with parchment paper, form clusters using about 60 ml (¼ cup) of the mixture for each.

4. Refrigerate for 1 to 2 hours before serving.

Did you know?

What is cardamom?
Native to India, this plant is in the same family as ginger and turmeric and grows in about thirty different varieties. The one we know best is green cardamom, which also happens to be the most flavourful. It can be purchased in powder, seed or pod form (we prefer the latter for a more pronounced taste). Its aroma hovers somewhere between lemon and eucalyptus and can be used in both sweet and savoury dishes. Infused as a tea, this spice is also great for digestion!

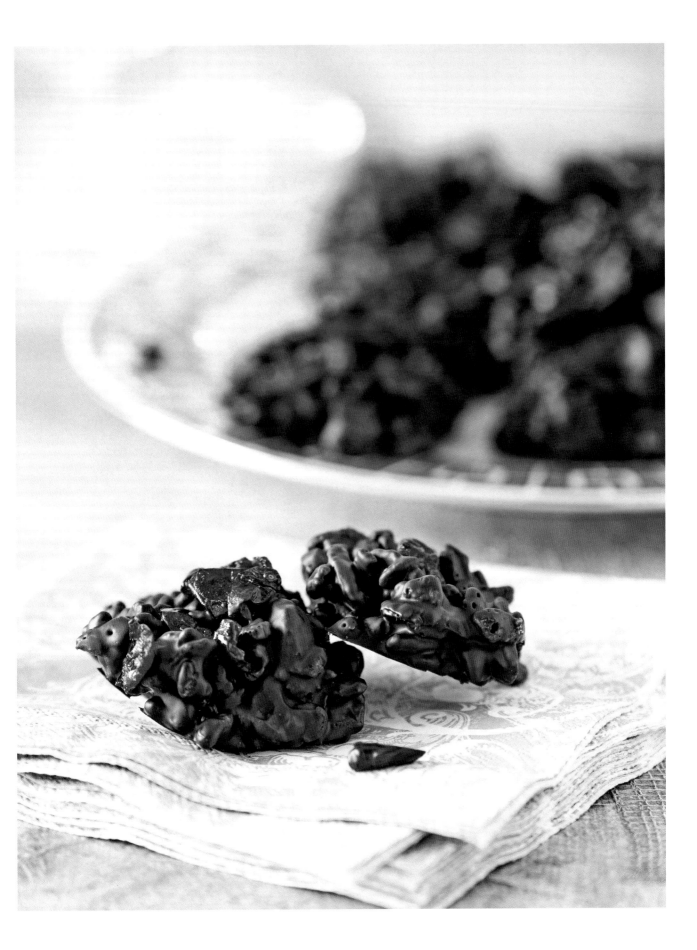

Chocolate and Red Kidney Bean Brownies

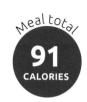

Meal total
91
CALORIES

125 ml (½ cup) red kidney beans, rinsed and drained

45 ml (3 tbsp) butter or non-hydrogenated margarine

90 g dark chocolate (70%), cut into pieces

60 ml (¼ cup) sugar

2 eggs

80 ml (⅓ cup) unbleached, all-purpose flour

60 ml (¼ cup) walnuts, chopped

Prep time **15 minutes**

Cook time **12 minutes**

Serves **16**

PER SERVING	
Calories	91
Protein	2 g
Fat	5 g
Carbohydrates	9 g
Fibre	1 g
Iron	1 mg
Calcium	10 mg
Sodium	9 mg

1. Preheat the oven to 180°C (350°F).

2. Puree the red kidney beans in a food processor.

3. Place the butter and 60 g of the dark chocolate in a microwave-safe bowl. Microwave for about 1 minute on high heat. Add the sugar and mix well.

4. Add the eggs one at a time, mixing thoroughly after each addition. Mix in the bean puree.

5. Gradually stir in the flour. Add the nuts.

6. Grease a 20 cm (8 in) square baking dish and pour in the batter. Bake for 12 to 15 minutes, until a toothpick inserted into the centre comes out clean.

7. Remove the dish from the oven and let cool completely.

8. While the brownies are cooling, melt the rest of the chocolate in a bain-marie water bath or the microwave.

9. Remove the brownies from the dish and cut into 16 squares. Use a spoon to drizzle melted chocolate over each square.

Recipe by Ève Godin, nutritionist

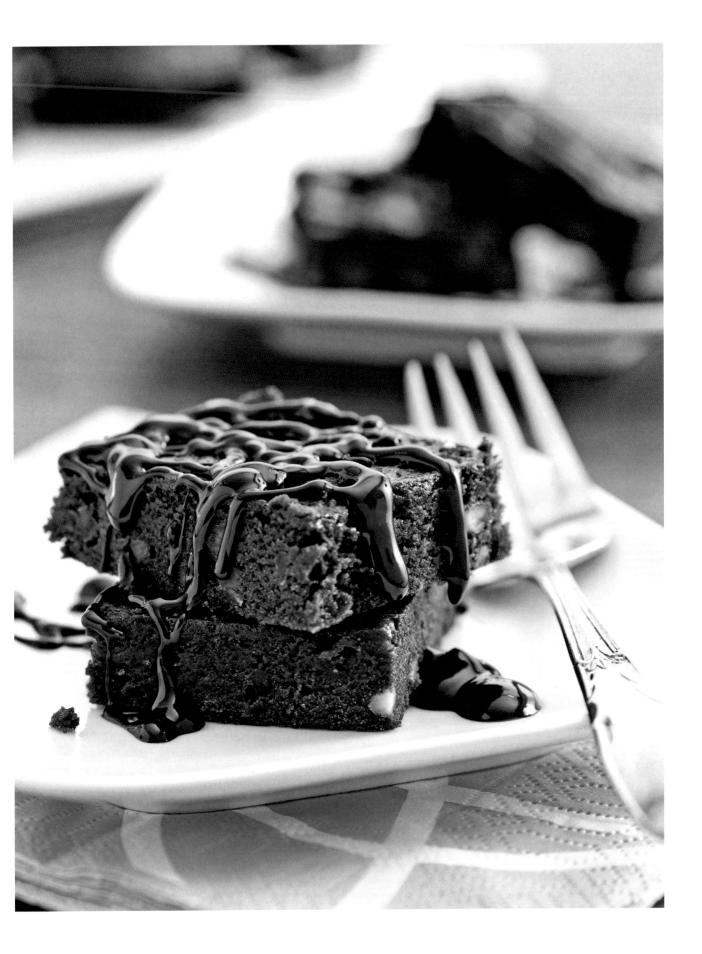

Baked Doughnuts

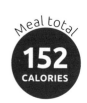

Meal total
152
CALORIES

450 g (1 lb) potatoes

30 ml (2 tbsp) vanilla extract

500 ml (2 cups) sugar

125 ml (½ cup) butter, lightly melted

1.75 litre (7 cups) flour

30 ml (2 tbsp) baking powder

500 ml (2 cups) 1% milk

180 ml (¾ cup) maple syrup (optional)

Prep time **45 minutes**

Cook time **10 minutes**

Yields **40 to 45 doughnuts**

PER SERVING	
Calories	152
Protein	3 g
Fat	2 g
Carbohydrates	30 g
Fibre	1 g
Iron	1 mg
Calcium	26 mg
Sodium	35 mg

1. Preheat the oven to 180°C (350°F).

2. Peel the potatoes and cut into cubes. Place in a pot of cold water and bring to a boil. Cook until tender, drain and puree. Let cool slightly on the counter, and then refrigerate to cool completely.

3. Place the cooled pureed potatoes, vanilla, sugar and melted butter in a bowl. Stir until evenly mixed.

4. In another bowl, mix the flour with the baking powder. Pour the dry ingredients into the potato mixture. Gradually stir in the milk. Mix until smooth.

5. Fill the cups of a doughnut pan two-thirds of the way with batter.

6. Bake for 10 minutes, or until a toothpick inserted into the centre of a doughnut comes out clean. Dip the warm doughnuts into maple syrup if desired.

Did you know?

Doughnuts can be baked in the oven

Who doesn't like treating themselves to doughnuts every once in a while? But don't overdo it—doughnuts are typically fried in oil, which means a significant increase in calories, not to mention guilt! You can bypass this problem with our recipe for oven-baked doughnuts that are every bit as decadent. The moment you pop them in the oven instead, the calorie count drops without compromising taste. You'll need a doughnut pan to make them. Pick one up at most kitchen stores.

Original recipe from the Délices d'Antan bakery in Berthierville, modified for the oven

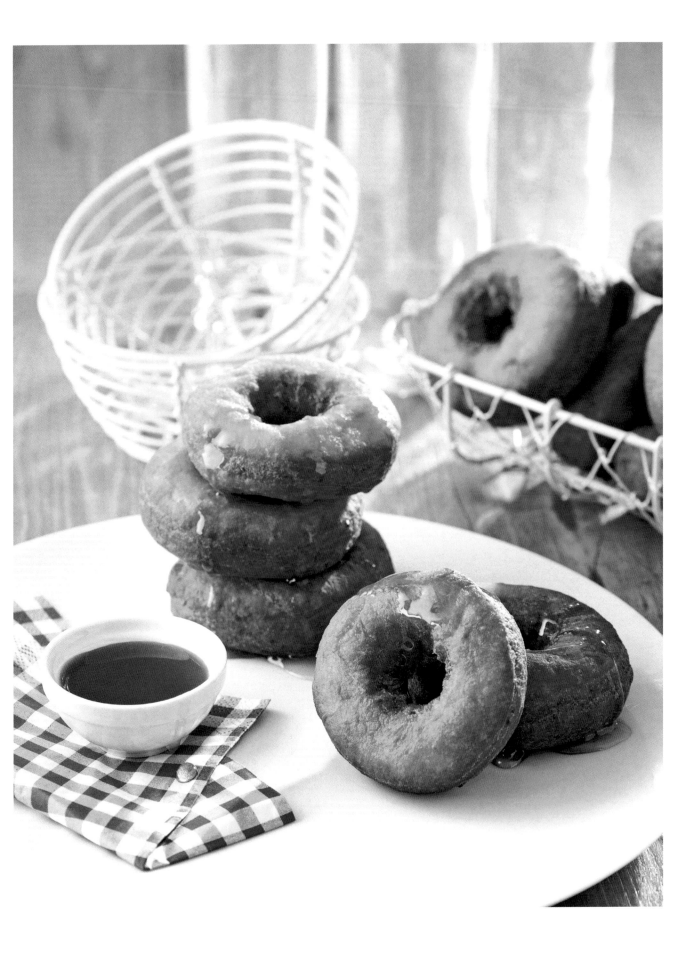

Chocolate Chip Cookies

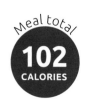

Meal total

102
CALORIES

125 ml (½ cup) whole wheat flour

250 ml (1 cup) quick-cooking oats

2.5 ml (½ tsp) baking soda

1 pinch salt

60 ml (¼ cup) softened butter

125 ml (½ cup) brown sugar

5 ml (1 tsp) vanilla extract

1 egg

50 g (1 ¾ oz) dark chocolate (70%), cut into pieces

Prep time **15 minutes**

Cook time **10 minutes**

Yields **16 cookies**

PER SERVING	
Calories	102
Protein	2 g
Fat	5 g
Carbohydrates	12 g
Fibre	1 g
Iron	1 mg
Calcium	13 mg
Sodium	58 mg

1. Preheat the oven to 190°C (375°F).

2. In a bowl, mix the flour with the oats, baking soda and salt.

3. Use an electric mixer to whip together the butter, brown sugar and vanilla until creamy. Whisk in the egg.

4. Gradually add the dry ingredients to the wet ingredients and stir until evenly mixed. Add the chocolate pieces and stir.

5. Form 16 balls of cookie dough with an ice cream scoop on a baking sheet lined with parchment paper. Leave 5 cm (2 in) of space between each cookie.

6. Bake for 10 to 12 minutes.

7. Remove the baking sheet from the oven and let cool on a rack.

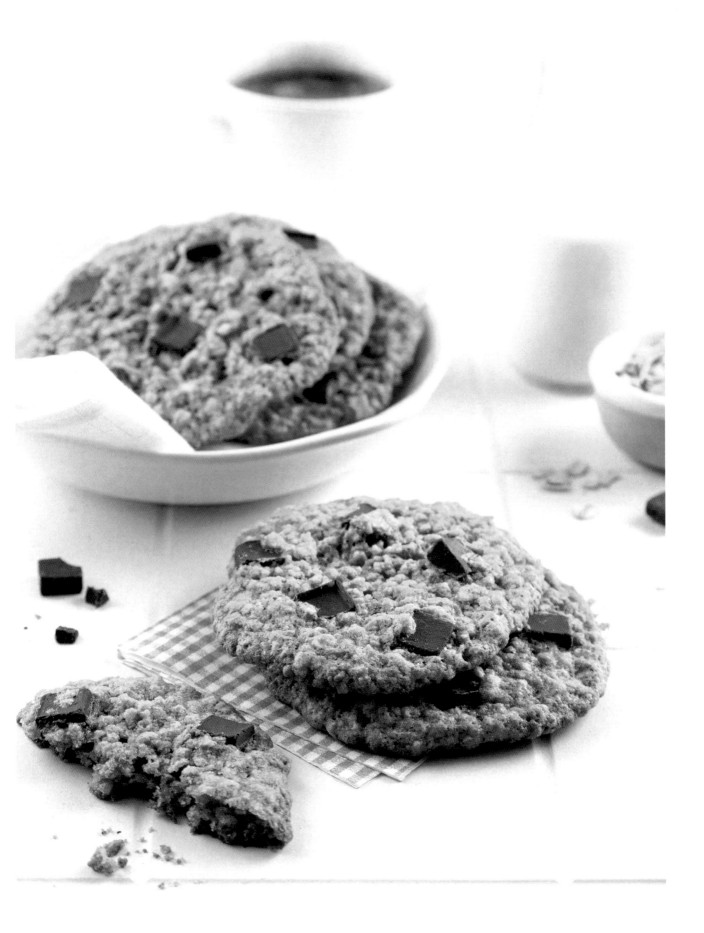

Recipes Index